"Zefiro Mellacqua's book is a cornerstone in contemporary transactional analysis for the understanding and treatment of the broad spectrum of psychotic disorders.

The Author provides a well-founded summary of Berne's transactional analysis theory and basic approach and then he develops his own innovative ideas which help understand psychosis in a new frame of reference, well connected to recent theories on relational traumas, and the importance of context (family, society, professional network) to cure psychotic patients.

At the core of Mellacqua's sensible approach we find the body as the unconscious theater of primal affective, sensory-motor relationships, very traumatic for the psychotic patient. The body may also communicate the starting point for a co-constructive search of meaning and direction which deeply involves both the therapist and the patient.

A close analysis of the transferential-countertransferential relationship and a review of specific Bernian techniques propose excellent methodological-technical tools for the clinical treatment.

The Author gives many interesting and touching examples taken from his clinical practice, which allow to better understand the nature of the relational processes that he has developed in his research on the treatment of psychotic patients.

Through Mellacqua's narratives we can capture his courage, passion, humanity and creativity that found his clinical work, and which seem to be an expression of the 'real philosophy of hope' that he sees at the core of Berne's revolutionary ideas: 'the hope of being able to share the almost ineffable human experience of being as "I" with a more or less large group of people, including those who are mentally suffering.'"

– **Maria Teresa Tosi**, PhD, Licensed Psychotherapist, TSTA, Past-President European Association of Transactional Analysis

"This book is a must read for anyone working with, or touched by, the unfathomable experience of schizophrenia. Examining research findings, theoretical debates, and rich case illustrations through his lens as a transactional analyst, Mellacqua enriches, and transforms, both our understanding of the phenomena he investigates and of the theory he draws on. Through the book, schizophrenia comes to light and to life as a deeply relational phenomenon, and even an avenue to examine the broader question of how selves emerge—or vanish or get fragmented—from bodies in relationships. Mellacqua's gifted writing humanizes the suffering of mental illness without romanticizing it. He combines the observations of an astute clinician, the erudition of a seasoned scholar, the finesse of an acute theorist, and the sensitivity of a poetic writer into a volume of exceptional clarity and humanity. This book's theories, like its stories, are an invitation to relate and examine relating. Both help approach, rather than dismiss, the uniqueness of selves longing, and failing, to do just that."

– **Gianpiero Petriglieri**, MD, Associate Professor of organisational behaviour, INSEAD

"In this book Zefiro Mellacqua takes us on a rigorous intellectual journey, tracing the origins and application of the theory of transactional analysis. This book is written with eloquence and style as Mellacqua outlines the original TA paradigm, faithfully following Berne's inspirational theories of the function and structure of ego states alongside his study of phenomenology. Mellacqua details the source of Berne's theories referring in some detail to the influence of psychoanalysis with particular attention to Paul Federn, Edward Weiss and Roland Fairbairn. It is a fascinating account of how transactional analysis moves away from the static and fixed entity of Freud's theory of ego by describing ego states as representing lived experiences in the present moment which, upon examination, may reflect archaic experiences and/or introjected messages from the past. In reading Mellacqua's narrative it becomes clear how TA theory lends itself to multiple innovative expression.

Mellacqua's innovative application of TA brings us into the psychiatric arena with a specific focus on schizophrenia. In his case studies the author shows how he works humanely and thoughtfully with patients who suffer from severe mental conditions. Mellacqua's humanity is also located in the context of his psychological and phenomenological knowledge in addition to his research into the latest scientific findings on the developing mind. This book provides the academic context for analysing the condition of schizophrenia and, at the same time, we feel emotionally connected to the author and his patients when he describes his case studies and his sensitive reflections about his patients. For these reasons I think the book has the potential to be a creative and solid support for psychiatrists in modern day practice.

For the TA clinician this book will take us back to the origins of Berne's thinking. It will be indispensable for trainees wishing to understand the structure of ego state theory for in his clarity of language Mellacqua reminds us of the potential for in depth exploration of the psyche alongside the practicality inherent in Berne's theoretical models. In particular this book will be an inspirational text for all clinicians within the profession of psychiatry who work alongside patients who suffer from schizophrenia. Mellacqua brings a depth of integrated intelligence and thus we are invited to engage with live patients, with a real doctor working patiently, reflectively, knowledgeably and with great sensitivity and empathy. The case studies are, for me, a testimony to the power for potent clinical practice working with patients who have serious mental health conditions."

– **Helena Hargaden**, DPsych, MSc, TSTA, Relational Transactional
Analyst, UKCP Registered Integrative Psychotherapist

TRANSACTIONAL ANALYSIS OF SCHIZOPHRENIA

In *Transactional Analysis of Schizophrenia: The Naked Self*, Zefiro Mellacqua presents a full assessment of the relevance and value of transactional analysis in understanding, conceptualizing, and treating schizophrenia in contemporary clinical settings.

Opening with a review of Eric Berne's ideas, Mellacqua applies theory to the understanding and psychotherapeutic treatment of people suffering from first-episode schizophrenia and to those already living with more long-lasting psychotic levels of self-disturbance. The chapters address a series of crucial methodological themes, including the need for both intensive and extensive analytic sessions; the therapist's tolerance of uncertainty and not knowing; the informative quality of both therapist's and patient's embodiment(s); the emergence of the transference-countertransference relationship; the link between silent transactions and unconscious communication; dream analysis; and the value of regular supervisions. Mellacqua's approach incorporates meetings with family and caregivers, as well as emphasizing multidisciplinary work with patients in a variety of settings, such as in hospitals, outpatient clinics, and psychiatric home treatment. The book is illustrated with engaging clinical case studies throughout, which illuminate the schizophrenic experience and provide examples of how these tools can be used to help patients.

Transactional Analysis of Schizophrenia demonstrates how those who suffer from acute schizophrenia, especially those at their very first episode of psychosis, can make an effective recovery and live a satisfying life through the therapeutic application of transactional analysis. It will be essential reading for transactional analysts, psychodynamically oriented psychotherapists, psychologists, psychiatrists, nurses, social workers, academics, and all mental health professionals working with people suffering from schizophrenic psychoses.

Zefiro Mellacqua is a psychiatrist and transactional analyst. He is a former researcher at the Institute of Psychiatry, King's College London, and psychiatrist with Lambeth Home Treatment Team, South London & Maudsley NHS Trust, UK. He is now leading the first Home Treatment Team for the Cantonal Sociopsychiatric Organization, Ticino, Switzerland.

INNOVATIONS IN TRANSACTIONAL ANALYSIS: THEORY AND PRACTICE

Series Editor: William F. Cornell

This book series is founded on the principle of the importance of open discussion, debate, critique, experimentation, and the integration of other models in fostering innovation in all the arenas of transactional analytic theory and practice: psychotherapy, counseling, education, organizational development, health care, and coaching. It will be a home for the work of established authors and new voices.

Titles in the series:

https://www.routledge.com/Innovations-in-Transactional-Analysis-Theory-and-Practice/book-series/INNTA

TRANSACTIONAL ANALYSIS OF SCHIZOPHRENIA

The Naked Self

Zefiro Mellacqua

Routledge
Taylor & Francis Group

LONDON AND NEW YORK

First published 2021
by Routledge
2 Park Square, Milton Park, Abingdon, Oxon OX14 4RN

and by Routledge
52 Vanderbilt Avenue, New York, NY 10017

Routledge is an imprint of the Taylor & Francis Group, an informa business

British Library Cataloguing-in-Publication Data
A catalogue record for this book is available from the British Library

Library of Congress Cataloging-in-Publication Data
Names: Mellacqua, Zefiro, author.
Title: Transactional analysis of schizophrenia : the naked self / Zefiro
Mellacqua.
Description: Milton Park, Abingdon, Oxon ; New York, NY : Routledge,
2020. | Includes bibliographical references and index.
Identifiers: LCCN 2020007489 (print) | LCCN 2020007490 (ebook) |
ISBN 9780367148409 (hardback) | ISBN 9780367148423 (paperback) |
ISBN 9780429053566 (ebook)
Subjects: LCSH: Schizophrenia. | Transactional analysis. | Psychotherapy.
Classification: LCC RC514 .M427 2020 (print) | LCC RC514 (ebook) |
DDC 616.89/8--dc23
LC record available at https://lccn.loc.gov/2020007489
LC ebook record available at https://lccn.loc.gov/2020007490

ISBN: 978-0-367-14840-9 (hbk)
ISBN: 978-0-367-14842-3 (pbk)
ISBN: 978-0-429-05356-6 (ebk)

Typeset in Times New Roman
by Taylor & Francis Books

TO CATERINA

CONTENTS

LIST OF FIGURES

ON BURROUGHS' WORK

The method must be purest meat
and no symbolic dressing,
actual visions & actual prisons
as seen then and now.

Prisons and visions presented
with rare descriptions
corresponding exactly to those
of Alcatraz and Rose.

A naked lunch is natural to us,
we eat reality sandwiches.
But allegories are so much lettuce.
Don't hide the madness.

Allen Ginsberg – San Jose, 1954

LIST OF CASES

ABBREVIATIONS

Key for author ego state abbreviations

P_0 — The internalized representation of the "Other as the environment" that is contacted by the emergent self (C_0) during intrauterine life and the very early stages of the infant's development

P_1 — The internal object representation containing the internalization of early object relations of the child with significant others (mother, father, caregivers, and anyone acting *in loco parentis*) during late infancy and early childhood

P_{1+} — The good object as the result of P_1 splitting and experienced by the developing child in terms of either good-enough or idealized primary relations with significant others

P_{1-} — The bad object as the result of P_1 splitting and being experienced by the developing child in terms of traumatic (persecutory, abusive etc.), intolerable, and demonized primary relations with significant others

P_2 — The Parent ego state consisting of conscious, preconscious, nonconscious, and unconscious cocreated experiences of the Other within (including the environment and real significant others) at different stages of self-development, but also as the container of the person in the world (i.e., society, culture, religion, etc.)

A_0 — The earliest sense of self resulting from the infant's experience of the mutual interaction with a self-regulating other

A_1 — The verbal, intersubjective and protoreflective self that represents the child's creative attempt to make sense of himself or herself, significant others, and the world based on his or her C_1 and P_1 experiences

A_2 — The Adult ego state consisting of conscious, preconscious, nonconscious, unconscious cocreated, and integrating experiences of the self in the here-and-now relationship with others and external reality

C_0 The emergent self containing the infant's bodily affective states that include the sense of being contacted by the "Other as environment" (P_0)

C_1 The core self or the embodied self coinciding with the Somatic Child and representing the tissue level of human experience and early bodily affective processes

C_2 The Child ego state as the whole self consisting of conscious, preconscious, nonconscious, and unconscious relational needs that not only result from C_1, A_1, P_1 and experiences but also continue throughout existence as a universal aspect of being human and therefore shaping self-identity

FOREWORD

William F. Cornell

ANISHA: I have my books, everything that is most dear to me.

ZEFIRO: And perhaps that's why the other evening when I got in from work I thought about that book by Tagore.

ANISHA: Hungry Stones, Anisha added quietly.

ZEFIRO: Precisely ... I saw something special in that title ... something to do with you, I think.

ANISHA: Really? she said to me curiously. And then she added, What do you mean?

ZEFIRO: I was thinking about your situation today ... I mean about your existential condition as well as the situation you're living in these days.

ANISHA: And what do you think?

ZEFIRO: Well, perhaps it's not a thought ... it's more an image of you ... yes, an image of you, but also of you and me here in this room like hungry stones, hungry stones, hungry for something.

ANISHA: Well, you can't judge a book by its cover. Silence.

ZEFIRO: Well said. But perhaps that's exactly what I'm trying to ask you: If you wish to open a page of your story, if you agree to brush the dust off the book of your life and share something personal with me.

What is it like to meet with a patient who long ago slammed shut the book, the stories, the memories, the longings, and the meanings of their life in a desperate attempt to simply remain alive? What is asked of us as mental health professionals to meet and work with people whose psyches have fragmented and retreated from engagement with the world as others prefer to know it? In *The Naked Self,* Zefiro Mellacqua brings alive his encounters with patients diagnosed as schizophrenic. He invites us to enter the world of psychotic defenses as he seeks to reach through to the core of patients that have been so long alienated from safe and enlivening contact with others. There are many interchanges Zefiro shares in the pages of this book that I could have chosen to begin this preface. I chose this one because it conveys a quiet and yet unmistakable longing on the part of Anisha and demonstrates Zefiro's clearly signaled respect for Anisha's right to make choices as to if and how to share something personal with him, to brush off the dust in his presence.

Zefiro insists that we don't hide the madness, and in his insistence, he speaks to professionals and patients alike. In so much of contemporary psychotherapy and psychiatry there are efforts to blunt, to hide, to turn away from madness. *The Naked Self* insists that we look, that we engage, that we listen, that we seek to grasp the meanings of forms of self experience and communication that have come to be cut off from the Other. How do we engage with a psyche that has long been in retreat?

Zefiro grounds his understanding and approach to schizophrenic patients within the theory and methodology of contemporary transactional analysis. In so doing, he opens the book with a chapter that brilliantly re-presents the groundbreaking ideas of Eric Berne through a contemporary lens. This is the single best accounting and reflection of the core of Berne's work that I have ever read.

I write this preface having worked as a psychotherapist in community mental health and private practice for 45 years, a period of time that has witnessed the systematic dismantling of humane, in-depth psychiatric and therapeutic services. Here in the US a group of mental health professionals have banded together as the Psychotherapy Action Network in an effort to challenge the collapse of meaningful mental health care:

> There is a deeply troubling trend in psychotherapy training and policy that emphasizes a view of emotional distress as a disease. This trend leads to factoring out the importance of relationships, categorizing human problems mainly in terms of symptoms or superficial forms of diagnosis, and viewing medication and short-term, manualized, or automated treatments as first-line remedies. These policies and practices undermine the core elements of successful mental health treatment, serving the commercial needs of Big Pharma and health insurance companies ahead of the needs of individuals and families.
>
> (Psychotherapy Action Network, 2019)

Zefiro Mellacqua articulates a position and a methodology that breathes life and meaning back into the treatment of these desperate states of mind, and being so often labeled as "schizophrenic". The theory and methodology that frames this book is that of transactional analysis, offering a perspective that is also well-informed by the history of psychiatry and influenced by contemporary object relations and relational models. In Zefiro's own words:

> The suffering of the ego in schizophrenia is thus a suffering that always occurs with the Other, regardless of the material presence of that Other in the patient's actual life. Schizophrenia shows how the Other is primarily the real parent (or a substitute) who has from the

earliest periods of development shirked on many occasions, and for a sufficiently long time, the onerous task of facilitating the young person's psychological as well as biological birth.

The psychotherapeutic engagement with "schizophrenic" patients is the opportunity for the new psychological birth and growth, often for both parties involved (this work does not leave the therapist unchanged). The central and compelling position that Zefiro articulates and demonstrates throughout these pages is that psychotic breakdowns are understandable and meaningful from within patients' familial and social contexts and are best treated within those contexts. Schizophrenic patients are not to be treated in isolation from family and other social supports. He brings a relentlessly humane perspective to the treatment of schizophrenia, as beautifully illustrated when he writes directly to those suffering from schizophrenia:

Do not fear medication as long as it is prescribed by someone who is caring for you as a person. Always give yourself a good dose of art and music. Walk in nature. Learn, if you don't already, to love animals.

ACKNOWLEDGMENTS

I would like to express my deepest gratitude first and foremost to all my patients, as this book could not have been conceived without them. I have been moved and transformed over time, on both a professional and more personal level, by their mental and bodily pain, their existential anguish, but also their resilience, their honesty, their courage and their hope. They have allowed me to gradually come closer to their almost ineffable suffering, teaching me how to explore and find meaning in their predicaments, to listen mindfully to our speaking bodies, to value the time spent together during often very long sessions, and to experience a vital connectedness to one another. I have also felt immensely privileged to have been able to meet their families and caregivers on many occasions, either in their homes or in my office. They have generously shared with me their emotions, doubts, reflections, and their own stories.

All clinical cases in the book have been disguised and anonymized to protect the confidentiality of patients and their caregivers, but my actual encounters, transactional dialogues and non-verbal interactions with them have been faithfully preserved to make the clinical material applicable to most therapists dealing with similar therapeutic challenges.

In particular, two chapters of this book, namely Chapter 3 and Chapter 4, contain entire passages taken from a seminal paper, "Beyond symbiosis", originally published in the *Transactional Analysis Journal*, 2014, 44(1), 1–23. Also Chapter 2 has just been accepted for publication in the *Transactional Analysis Journal* and it will be published in April 2020.

My gratitude goes to the editors of the journal and their publishers, who have generously granted me their permission to use parts of previous papers here.

This journey, however, would not even have been possible without meeting and developing a very long-standing professional and personal relationship with Pietro Petriglieri. He was Professor of Anatomy at the University of Catania (Sicily) where I trained both as a doctor and psychiatrist. He was an extraordinarily brilliant and humane teacher, and was also a neurologist, psychiatrist and transactional analysis practitioner himself. It was he who introduced me for the very first time to the work and life of Eric Berne, the founder of transactional analysis. Right at the beginning of my medical training, Prof Petriglieri gathered together a group of highly motivated medical students, of which I was one from 2001 to 2006, with the explicit aim of helping us deal with our difficult emotions and struggles in preparing for written and oral exams. However, our weekly encounters soon turned into a group therapy. I considered myself fortunate to have met him during this troubled period of my life when I was only a second-year medical student dealing with both personal and educational struggles. Pietro Petriglieri later became one of my first analysts and supervisor in my early days as a trainee in psychiatry and psychotherapy.

His sudden and unexpected death in 2016 was too soon followed by the passing of my beloved uncle Tonio – their loss left me with a deep sense of both solitude and gratitude at the same time. Without them I could not have imagined my life being as enriched and meaningful as it has been so far.

I am also deeply grateful to numerous colleagues as well as training and supervising analysts of the international transactional analysis community for providing me with the opportunity to present and discuss the ideas in this book at conferences and clinical seminars over the last few years. I would particularly like to offer my thanks to: William Cornell, Michael Landaiche, Helena Hargaden, Jo Stuthridge, Birgitta Heiller, James R. Allen, Pietro Petriglieri, Gianpiero Petriglieri, Raffaella Leone Guglielmotti, Giorgio Cavallero, Loredana Paradiso, Antonella Liverano, Maria Gioia Milizia, Maria Teresa Tosi, Silvia Attanasio Romanini, and Alessandra Pierini.

Special thanks go specifically to all the senior trainers and colleagues at the Auximon Institute of Transactional Analysis in Rome where I trained as a therapist.

Profound thanks also go to the wonderful group of Romanian colleagues, Marina Vasile, Alexandra Gheorghe, Delia Codreanu, Diana Deaconu, Lucia Ionas, Nicoleta Gheorghe, who all carefully read and commented upon every single paragraph of the initial paper on the same subject: they have enormously enriched and challenged my thinking about a series of issues that later found their way into this book.

I would also like to remember Prof Antonino Petralia, a highly dedicated forensic psychiatrist at the University of Catania, who positively challenged my clinical thinking over the years when I used to travel from Sicily to Rome to attend transactional analysis training in psychotherapy, and who supported my intention to improve my clinical skills and psychiatric training abroad.

There are many others to thank for their incredible support and encouragement: the many colleagues and friends I met (or re-found) during my time in London between 2008 and 2015. These mostly include highly distinguished clinicians, professors, researchers, and psychotherapists from the field of first-episode psychosis. I would particularly like to mention:

- Prof Paola Dazzan for accepting my very first application to work with her team at the Department of Psychological Medicine at the Institute of Psychiatry, King's College London, and to whom I owe a tremendous debt of gratitude for first introducing me to the fascinating world of neuroimaging of first-episode schizophrenia, and for having masterfully guided me through the arduous work of clinical research with patients.
- Prof Robin Murray, Prof Anthony David and Prof Craig Morgan to whom go my sincere thanks for their elevating inspiration and encouraging guidance throughout my research fellowship in the field of psychosis at the Institute of Psychiatry, King's College London.
- Dr Larry Rifkin, consultant psychiatrist with the Lambeth Home Treatment Team, part of the South London and Maudsley NHS Foundation Trust, and senior clinical lecturer at the Institute of Psychiatry, Psychology and Neuroscience, to whom I am immensely grateful for our joint home visits in Lambeth, for his extraordinary clinical mentorship and regular supervisions of very complex clinical cases.
- All the nurses, occupational therapists, support workers, clinical psychologists, team managers, social workers, approved mental health professionals (AMHPs), honorary consultants, visiting colleagues, trainees and students with whom I had the privilege to work during my years with the Lambeth Home Treatment Team (2010–2015), and from whom I learned the most about how to collaboratively both care for and cure people in the midst of a psychotic breakdown.
- Rekha Dave, a senior nurse and manager at Balppa House in the heart of Elephant and Castle in London, who trusted my clinical expertise enough to give me the opportunity to see patients for psychotherapy sessions outside of my NHS working hours late in the evenings and during weekends.
- The special group of highly dedicated and eclectic clinicians, as well as exceptionally enthusiastic researchers, colleagues and friends, all from Italy, in particular Marianna Ciancio, Felice Loi, Stefania Bonaccorso, Martino Belvederi Murri, Manuela Russo, Ilenia Pampaloni, Francesca Ducci, Sara Pozzoli, Simona Stilo, and later on Costanza Vecchio, Vincenzo Perri and Carlo Negro for all the fun, great meals and beautiful times we shared together along the way, and for our continuing friendship.

Indeed, London was the place where I developed a deeper understanding of myself and my patients, thanks in the first place to my analysis and supervision with Helena Hargaden, towards whom I feel indebted to this day.

I have always been interested in psychoanalysis, phenomenology and philosophy, and I was fortunate enough to be able to attend a series of lectures on these subjects at the Tavistock Centre, University College London, the Freud Museum, and at the Institute of Psychiatry, Psychology and Neuroscience (IoPPN). During those years I became an avid reader, besides Berne, of various psychoanalytic authors such as Paul Federn, Wilfred Bion, Donald Winnicott,

Jacques Lacan, Didier Anzieu, Esther Bick, Herbert Rosenfeld, Harold Searles, Gaetano Benedetti, Luc Ciompi and more contemporary analysts such as Paul Williams, Diego Napolitani, Salomon Resnik, Antonino Ferro, Franco De Masi, Christopher Bollas, and William Cornell.

Some of their ideas and deeply humane contributions to the understanding and treatment of psychosis have filtered into this work in many, sometimes unpredictable, ways.

I also owe much to my translator Laura Massey, who with professional determination, growing enthusiasm, and a deep sense of how language conveys meaning, translated most of the actual book, which was originally written in Italian.

Additional thanks go unequivocally to Robin Fryer, editor of the *Transactional Analysis Journal*, who kindly reviewed my first article on schizophrenia and later saw this book through to its conclusion with meticulous editing and energy. Her extraordinary contribution and dedication helped me refine some crucial ideas and expand on some important themes of the book by keeping in mind the reader's perspective.

A very special expression of my gratitude must go to my editor William Cornell for his encouragement and generous support, for his genuine appreciation of my writings over the years, and for even honoring me with the Preface to this book. His deeply inspiring clinical work and his consistent receptiveness and responsiveness continue to be intellectually and emotionally nurturing. He helped me shape the book while giving me the opportunity to find my own voice.

I thank Susannah Frearson, Editor at Routledge (UK), for taking on this book and to Heather Evans, Senior Editorial Assistant at Taylor and Francis Group, for her comments and editorial assistance.

I am indebted to many more people, but I am especially grateful to my family for their continued love, trust, incredible sacrifices, and encouragement in both good times and bad. I have had wonderful personal support during my life from my parents and my sister Eufrasia, my grandparents, as well as my uncles and my aunt who have believed in me and helped me in every possible way.

Finally there are no words to adequately express my profound gratitude to my wife Maria for the grace with which she made room in her life for my many long weekend hours of work, late nights and even later dinners. She both generously and lovingly accepted my preoccupation with this book, being incredibly understanding and supportive throughout the whole writing process. She is a true listener and a precious partner, who has been able to bring balance, joy, and constant hopeful vision to my work and, most importantly, to our family life.

And last but not least, I dedicate this book to my wonderful daughter Caterina to whom I owe, together with my wife, the inestimable gift of parenthood with its profound joys and concerns, responsibilities, wonders and hopes in addition to the most delightful love and fun.

CREDIT LINES

Chapters 3 and 4 contain passages from Zefiro Mellacqua's (2014) article "Beyond symbiosis: The role of primal exclusions in schizophrenic psychosis," *Transactional Analysis Journal*, 44(1), 1–23, used with permissions.

Chapter 2 appears as the (2020) article "When a mind breaks down: A brief history of efforts to understand schizophrenia," *Transactional Analysis Journal*, 50(2), 117–129, used with permissions.

INTRODUCTION

Ode to the invisible man

H. G. Wells's science fiction novel *The Invisible Man* was published in 1897 and has had an appreciable cultural influence on comics, cinema, television, theater, and pop music—in particular, the song of the same name on the album *The Miracle* released in 1989 by British rock band Queen. In it the protagonist, Griffin, uses his own ingenuity to acquire the power of invisibility. In order to be invisible, however, circumstances force Griffin to be almost totally naked for most of the time.

Of the countless reflections the novel calls on us to make, there is one, in particular, that pertains to the strange, I would almost say disconcerting and sometimes even violent reaction of human beings toward the different, the grotesque, the mysterious, the unknown, the mad.

My book is essentially an attempt to reframe this reflection within the clinical domain and, in particular, through the analysis of what can be thought of as the most pervasive and disturbing of mental afflictions: schizophrenia. I have elected to do this by reconstructing relevant excerpts from my clinical work as a psychiatrist and transactional analyst practicing in London between 2010 and 2015 with people suffering from first-episode schizophrenia and with those already living with more long-lasting psychotic levels of self-disturbance.

But, for the moment, I want to return to Wells's novel. In it, the character's invisibility is portrayed as a strenuous search and certainly not as a condition with a definitive endpoint. In fact, despite being invisible, Griffin's naked body betrays his very invisibility. One might say that his bodily self, even when rendered completely invisible to others, continues to leave indirect traces of his irreducible corporality (physicality): through its movements, odors, the fact that it feels cold and pain like any other human body.

Without a natural and visible outer casing such as that provided by the human skin, the invisible man is exposed to a condition that is far worse than the feared visibility, namely, a progressive estrangement from his inner self and from others:

"I could not go abroad in snow—it would settle on me and expose me. Rain, too, would make me a watery outline, a glistening surface of a man—a bubble. And fog—I should be like a fainter bubble in a fog, a surface, a greasy glimmer of humanity. Moreover, as I went abroad—in the London air—I gathered dirt about my ankles, float-ing smuts and dust upon my skin. I did not know how long it would be before I should become visible from that cause also. But I saw clearly it could not be for long.

"But you begin now to realise," said the Invisible Man, "the full disadvantage of my condition. I had no shelter—no covering—to get clothing was to forego all my advantage, to make myself a strange and terrible thing. I was fasting; for to eat, to fill myself with unas-similated matter, would be to become grotesquely visible again."

(Wells, 2017 [1897], p. 126)

The end of Griffin actually begins with his body decomposing, which leads to a progressive alteration in his state of consciousness and then to madness, ending finally with his death at the hands of a mob. The level of madness attained by Griffin calls to mind—albeit through different ways from those of science fiction—the particular fragmentation of the self of the person with schizophrenia.

This madness derives from the impossibility of the human mind to over-come the sensory paradigm that, in this specific case, produces vision (though the same would also be true for the other senses), the faculty able to act as a human being's intermediary between the experience of being seen (i.e., recognized) by others and the construction of a personal sense of identity, between appearing and being. And so, we can hear the anguish of a psychotic patient echoed in Griffin's despairing cry when he exclaims:

"I wish you'd keep your fingers out of my eye," said the aerial voice, in a tone of savage expostulation. "The fact is, I'm all here—head, hands, legs, and all the rest of it, but it happens I'm invisible. It's a confounded nuisance, but I am."

(Wells, 2017 [1897], p. 40)

The tragedy of the schizophrenic, like that of Griffin, comes to coincide with the fragmentation of the experience of self and, ultimately, with alienation. The particular estrangement of the schizophrenic can be classified into a number of different forms on the clinical level. The first is a way of perceiving others and external reality as foreign bodies, alien to one's self, if not even as an actual threat to one's integrity, as occurs in cases of severe paranoid schizophrenia. The second condition, which is almost unbearable for the psychotic, is to perceive himself or herself and be perceived by others—including the therapist—as a multitude of sensory and bodily experiences without any internal coherence, as occurs in cases of disorganized schizophrenia. Third, in some cases, schizophrenic alienation is similar to the condition of a body that is apparently inert, suspended in time, even devoid of verbalizable experiences and therefore of a story to tell, as in extreme cases of obstinate mutism and immobility that can be observed in generally less common forms of catatonic schizophrenia.

This book examines in detail, from the perspective of transactional analysis, each of these conditions into which the self of the person with schizophrenia flows. This analysis necessarily includes the bodily self of the therapist, which is invariably immersed, often without the clinician's knowledge, in the same field of unconscious relationality that the patient with schizophrenia inhabits. Finding ourselves facing the fear of fragmentation of the experience of one's own self that the schizophrenic embodies, and at the same time powerfully induces in others, each of us—even mental health professionals—erects walls of suspiciousness; raises flags of hostility; creates barricades of scorn; digs underground tunnels of shame; hides in impenetrable forests of silence or, even worse, indifference; withdraws occasionally into the solitary strongholds of pharmacotherapy; gets lost in the distant labyrinths of intellectualism; and crosses boundless seas of solitude and hope not unlike those crossed by patients with schizophrenia in their strenuous attempt to preserve a vital core of their own self. To this vital self that is not immediately visible, often mute, dreamy, in some cases petrified and malodorous, bearer of wounds and scars as living memories of past traumas, yet resistant to the ineffable pain of alienation, I have given the name "the naked self." Readers are invited to meet it and recognize it not only in these pages but in their lives, in our own schizophrenic moments, which we find, not by chance, in our corporeity, in dreams, and, specifically, in the courageous and invaluable analytic and extra-analytic work with psychotic patients.

The reflections found in these pages are the fruit not only of often long and multiple clinical meetings with my schizophrenic patients but also of the opportunities (or not) I have had to actively engage with their families and caregivers. When these people were physically present and, more particularly, willing to join in the dialogue and engage, their suffering, questions, thoughts, silences, fears, shame, and hopes were often—and in some cases continue to be—mine too.

The learning and personal, as well as professional, growth that has resulted from my psychotherapeutic work with these patients and their loved and hated ones could not have progressed without the additional professional and human contributions made by my supervisors. A special mention of thanks to each of them can be found in the Acknowledgments, where the reader will also find additional anecdotal information about how this book came to be written.

My ultimate aim in writing this manuscript is to make visible and hopefully rich in existential meaning—specifically through the lens provided by Eric

Berne's transactional analysis and in line with his theoretical, methodological, and ethical principles—the not immediately visible and the invisible of schizophrenic suffering. I do this so that my—and, I believe, also your—clinical and human work aimed at understanding and treating this affliction can continue with even greater awareness, responsibility, dedication, and hope.

References

Queen (1989). The invisible man. On *The Miracle* [CD]. London: Parlophone.

Wells, H. G. (2017). *The invisible man*. London: HarperCollins. (Original work published 1897)

SPECIAL INTRODUCTION TO READERS WITH SCHIZOPHRENIA

These words are addressed to you, my invisible reader, my invisible person facing schizophrenia, and to those who are by your side, such as your family, possibly your partner, children, friends, teachers, colleagues, and anyone who truly cares about you and, at the same time, is deeply troubled and bewildered, just like you are, by such an almost ineffable yet unbearable suffering.

Hello, are you there? I know you are still there, listening, waiting, dealing with bodily discomforts, living through the chaos of present sensations, hiding away from people and from yourself. So, how are you now? How are you managing your days and nights? How are you dealing with your internal experiences? Can you trust your mind, your heart, your own body? Are you still wearing a sweater despite the hot weather? Are you wearing sunglasses even at night or indoors? Do you feel your head bursting sometimes? Are you constantly listening to music loudly in your earphones to drown out the voices in your head or to avoid the company of others? Have you found yourself laughing or shouting uncontrollably?

And what do external reality, the world, nature, and places look like to you? Have you been aggressive, physically or verbally, to anyone? Has anyone been physically or verbally aggressive to you? Are you carrying a knife to protect yourself? Have you harmed yourself? Are you still angry or sad or ashamed for what happened to you or to others because of your behavior? Do you look at yourself in the mirror from time to time? What do you see there? Does it scare you? Does it interest you in some way? And what are the reactions of others toward your strangeness? Can you bear it? Can they bear it? Is there anybody around you who is able to bear it? Even for a little while? Can you truly rely on someone else, besides yourself? Is this someone else next to you asking themselves similar questions, having the same fears, sharing or rejecting the same experiences you are wondering about? Do you talk to each other about these doubts, emotions, opinions, and beliefs? Do you really listen to each other? Do you do things together?

Are you able to cook for yourself? Are you eating healthily? Are you looking after your personal hygiene? Or do you need practical help? Can you sleep at night? Do you dream when you are asleep? Do you daydream? Do you have pets? How do you behave with them? Are you praying for your health? Or are you swearing under your breath? Can you trust medication? And can you trust a doctor (including a psychiatrist), a nurse, a psychologist, and any mental health professional who is there caring and willing to help you? Are there, actually, any of these people looking after you and your caregivers or at least trying to do so? And are you allowing them to help you or not? And if not, why not? And if yes, why?

If you are still wrestling with any of these questions, or if you are about to dismiss them because you are sick of them, or possibly because your thoughts are not that clear any more or are confounded by voices and by multiple odd sensations, then you may want to go through some other ideas, dialogues, stories, and dreams as first-hand lived experiences of psychosis and their respective therapeutic journeys as they are narrated in this book. I realize that some pages may sound too technical or distant from what you normally read. But some words or phrases, even simple ones, may actually speak directly to your mind, may warm your heart, may make you cry with pain and, possibly, with joy and hope, or they may simply make you wonder about yourself, about the nature of your symptoms and difficulties, about your past, about your actual life, and about your future. Or at least I hope so. I truly hope that you allow your self to come to light, to be visible and live your life more fully.

1

THE TRANSACTIONAL EGO IN CONTEMPORARY CLINICAL PRACTICE

Epistemological foundations and the legacy of Eric Berne's theory of ego states

Transactional analysis regards human subjectivity as a unique, unrepeatable set of ego states. In the view of the creator of transactional analysis, Eric Berne (1970), ego states are, in fact, "its foundation stones and its marks" in as much as "whatever deals with ego states is transactional analysis, and whatever overlooks them is not" (p. 223).

In the uninterrupted flow of each of our inner and relational lives, the ego is the part of the human personality that is able to observe itself, "much as the parts of the body can feel one other" (Berne, 1969 [1957], p. 87). Berne distinguished three parts within the ego, each of which is able, insofar as it is all one ego, to be aware of the others. These three parts are fundamental ways of existing, the result of the human experience of being and being in the world, a world that from the beginning of life is populated not only by a "me" and many "other-than-me" but also by an "us," by "many-Other(s)-within-me," and by a "me-through-the-Other(s)." In other words, there is no original "me" without a historical "Other" so that the "we," like the "me," inevitably carries a trace of the "Other."

Berne called the "me-through-the-Other(s)" the *Child* ego state—a kind of "residual infantile ego state of the adult person" (Weiss as cited in Berne, 1975b [1961], p. 19)—recalling how every individual carries inside him or her the child that was and continues to be in the present, as well as in the future, in relation to the important others of the past.

Another part of the ego is the *Parent*, or "the-Other(s)-within-me," a "psychic presence" (Weiss as cited in Berne 1975b [1961], p. 19) deriving from the internalization of parental figures or reference figures in *loco parentis*. These, over the course of the subject's past as well as throughout his or her life, are created, or not, through multiple and changing identifications and internalizations into normative and emotional authorities.

1

The *Adult* ego state, or the "me" (that is not the other), is the part of the personality that enables contact *between* the ego and the new other—also understood as environment and nature—thereby forming a "we." It is thanks to the Adult that the individual not only responsibly experiments with being a subjective ego with a history but accesses external reality, and primarily the psychological reality of the new other, with renewed curiosity, capturing the wonder and mystery of it in current experience—of both the here and now and the "not yet" (see Figure 1.1).

These three parts of the ego—Parent, Adult, and Child—operate within the healthy personality as discrete systems. Each is capable of operating both autonomously and together with the others, and has, on the one hand, its own internal organization and being, and on the other, is in continuous relationship with external reality.

The substance that makes an ego state is life that throbs with emotion, which is further expressed in thoughts and articulated in bodily experiences and visible behaviors. An ego state is, by Berne's definition, a consistently structured way of thinking, feeling, and behaving at any given moment. Moreover, as phenomenological realities, ego states are not "roles" (Berne, 1975b [1961], p. 33; 2008 [1964], p. 23) but living parts of the self with history and ever-evolving subjective experience. One could therefore say that ego states are innumerable but still related to each of the three parts of the ego that, according to the experience of psychological and social life, we call in transactional analysis Parent, Adult, and Child.

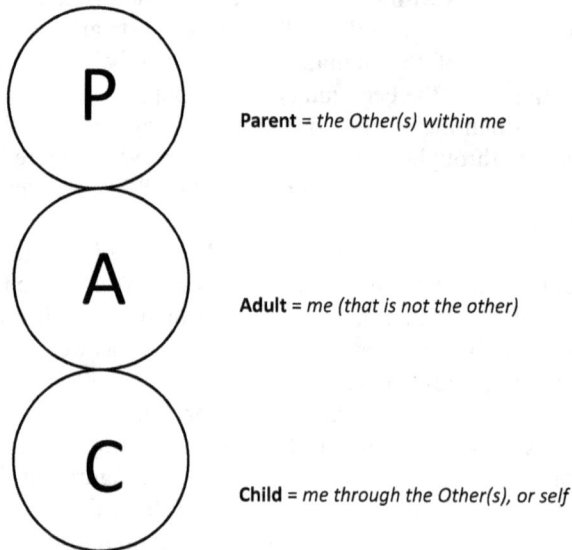

Parent = *the Other(s) within me*

Adult = *me (that is not the other)*

Child = *me through the Other(s), or self*

Figure 1.1 Ego states (adapted from Berne, 1975b [1961], p. 31)

The clinical and theoretical perspective adopted by Berne is marked by the influence from the 1940s and 1950s of the psychoanalytic psychology of the ego developed by Paul Federn (1953[1952]), Edoardo Weiss (1950), and Ronald Fairbairn (1952). In particular, the Bernean definition of ego state decisively contains the original contribution introduced by Federn (1953 [1952]) and Weiss (1950) into the analytical tradition as a phenomenological critique of Freud's vision of the ego as a psychic entity that originates from the id. For Federn, as for Berne, the ego is a phenomenological reality that can be experienced directly by the subject: "The ego is felt and known by the individual as a lasting or recurring continuity of the body and mental life in respect of time, space, and causality, and is felt and apprehended by him as a 'unity'" (Federn, 1953 [1952], p. 94). This formulation of the ego, originally produced by Federn, corresponds to the concept of ego state expressed by his greatest pupil, Edoardo Weiss (1950): "Every ego state is the actually experienced reality of one's mental and bodily ego with the contents of the lived-through period" (p. 141).

Furthermore, the theoretical perspective used by Berne regarding the tripartite idea of the ego—classified into Parent, Adult, and Child—found in Fairbairn's work (1952) is "one of the best heuristic bridges between transactional analysis and psychoanalysis" (Berne, 1975c [1972], p. 162). In fact, Fairbairn was the first to recognize a plural ego that is structured and differentiated—into a *central ego* (directed toward external relationships, especially if they are rewarding), a *libidinal ego* (linked to the search and hope for a relationship), and an *anti-libidinal ego* (linked to the hostility and rejection of relationships)—directly through more or less rewarding multiple relationships with real relational objects.

One could even say that Berne's theory, which is set out formally in *Transactional Analysis in Psychotherapy* (1975b [1961]), boosted and radicalized Fairbairn's thesis of the nonindivisibility of the ego, showing, rather, how the individual is populated by ego states on the inside (i.e., made up of internal objects that result from being constantly in relation to and identification with real, external others, the world, and surrounding nature).

Berne, following in the footsteps of the aforementioned authors, went further, boldly demonstrating four routes to forming knowledge—or diagnoses (from the Greek *dia-gnosis*, from διά "through" and γνωσις "knowledge", and therefore "to know through")—in a given moment of one's own or another's ego state and thereby meeting oneself as well as truly meeting the other in one's own uniqueness.

The first route to knowledge is observing behavior—one's own and other people's—in its myriad manifestations, such as body posture, gait, tone, volume and rhythm of the voice, breathing, vocabulary, gestures, and facial expression.

The second route to knowledge is social observation or the kind of behavioral response requested by the individual from the other during an interaction and vice versa. Social knowledge of an ego state is based on the assumption that one often forms a relationship starting from complementary or symmetrical ego states. For example, it is possible to work out if someone is in a Parent ego state by observing that his or her interlocutor is responding to the person from a Child ego state or from a Parent ego state in symmetrical competition.

The third way to recognize an ego state is by means of a historical (or psychobiographical) investigation of the person's traceable memories regarding the who and when of relational experiences from childhood and early adolescence with parental reference figures and significant others from the individual's past. Historical investigation facilitates an exploration of whether the ego state observed in the here and now is, in fact: (1) an expression of thoughts, emotions, and behaviors used by the reference parent(s) (Parent ego state); (2) inner experiences of the child that the person was in that particular historical moment (Child ego state); or (3) a response to the current situation (Adult ego state).

The fourth way to identify an ego state is through phenomenological exploration. More than the other ways, this route enables the greatest participation in the inner world of the other, introducing us and exposing us in all its intensity to the most distinctively subjective and idiosyncratic experience of the person in front of us. For example, a Child ego state or a Parent ego state is phenomenologically accessible when the subject does not simply remember but re-creates with all his or her expressive potency the cognitive, bodily-emotional, and relational experiences of a situation from his or her past and relives them in the present.

Berne (2008 [1964], p. 42) added to these means of knowing (or recognizing) ego states as observable psychological and social entities a description of how each part of the ego—Parent, Adult, and Child—can function in relation to the other parts (*influencing ego state*) and in social interaction with others (*active ego state*). In particular, in *What do you say after you say hello?*, Berne (1975c [1972], p. 32) showed in greater detail how the Parent can be described as *Nurturing Parent* (e.g., as provider of care, protection, and/or permission) or *Controlling Parent* (e.g., as a source of abuse, criticism, and/or prohibitions). On the other hand, the Child has also been classified by Berne (1975c [1972], p. 32) in descriptive terms such as *Adapted Child* (e.g., usually compliant toward parental or primary figures), *Rebellious Child* (e.g., openly hostile and rebellious toward regulatory others), and *Natural Child* (e.g., in tune with the person's own needs and acknowledged in respect of these by significant others).

Unlike the other parts of the ego, the Adult ego state did not have ascribed to it as many descriptive definitions by Berne. Instead, he attributed to and recognized in the Adult the unique possibility of a genuine approach to internal (one's own ego states) and external (ego states of others and the social world) contingent reality with all the cognitive, emotional, and

4

relational resources permitted to the Adult ego state by the biology of the individual's central and peripheral nervous system up to that moment in his or her development.[1]

Consequently, if the behavioral, social, historical, and phenomenological investigations lead to an actual presentation of an ego state ("Who am I?" "Who are you?" "Who is speaking, feeling, acting?"), then the description of the relational function of an ego state—as in the case of the Natural, Adapted, and Rebellious Child as well as the Nurturing and Controlling Parent—is, in fact, a phenomenal (i.e., behavioral) representation of it ("How am I?" "How are you?" "How am I speaking, feeling acting?" "How are you speaking, feeling, acting?")[2].

In essence, with the functional representation of ego states, Berne wanted not only to emphasize once again the observable behavioral aspects of each ego state but also to describe the type of function that an ego state plays in the ecology of the human mind, which is to maintain a sort of homeostasis of the subject's inner and relational (and therefore social) world.

Transactions: The mind in action

It is precisely in the acknowledgment of the existence of ego states within every personality that Berne showed us a new way of observing and understanding an encounter between two or more people. He deliberately chose the word *transaction* to show what is happening in a social exchange. It was not interaction or interpersonal connection or even relationship but transaction that was Berne's favored object and on which he focused. That was because transaction involves each individual engaging in something in every encounter, and, at the same time, something is exchanged, and what we get out of it is the reason each of us engages in it (Berne, 1975b [1961]).

With these as the premises, it is not surprising to find in Berne's writings diagrams and vectors that are means, and certainly not ends, for rendering not just a surprisingly creative and powerful vision of the intrapsychic and interpersonal worlds of the individual but for making this world understandable and accessible to the person himself or herself. Berne's revolution was, therefore, to have woven his own ideas about human subjectivity around a real philosophy of hope: the hope of being able to share the almost ineffable human experience of being an "I" with a more or less large group of people, including those who are mentally suffering.

The epistemological roots of this Bernean hope sink once again into the fertile soil of ego psychology, the central thesis of which is founded—starting from the work of Heinz Hartmann (1939), one of its greatest exponents—on the recognition of a core of the ego that is free from driving intrapsychic conflicts with their Freudian overtones. This part of the ego would consequently form an innate core of the personality, one that is able to develop in an independent way—unlike Freud's id—following precise neurophysiological bases and mediating, along the various phases of psychophysical development, the fragile connection of the individual with internal reality (intraegoic reality), his or her own body and those of others (intrabodily and interbodily reality), external relational reality (preobject relational world and interegoic reality), and the surrounding world and nature more generally.

These foundations of post-Freudian—or, as Berne wrote, para-Freudian—analytical knowledge converged in Berne's elaboration of the Adult ego state. He conceived of the Adult as a structure of the individual's personality that would be able to maintain areas (even if these are minimal, as in cases of serious psychopathology) that are notably free from both intrapsychic conflict and structural deficits. In this way, and also through the psychotherapeutic process, the person's Adult would become the part of the personality that is able to structure itself more and more extensively as an observing, self-reflective, self-analyzing, and integrating ego. In Berne's conception of the Adult ego state, there are echoes of the contemporary observations of Fenichel (as cited by Berne, 1977d [1966]) on "the division of the ego into an observing portion and an experiencing portion" (p. 293).

In other words, it is due to the operation of our psyche's Adult that, in Berne's view, a *transactional analysis proper* is possible. This involves analyzing the transactions between the egos of the various participants in a social encounter. Particularly in the clinical arena, this approach clearly retains its validity not only in a group setting but, given the plural nature of the ego, also in encounters between just two people, as, for example, in individual psychotherapy.

Since there would be no transactional analysis without a focus on the plural nature of the ego and the dimension of time—historical as well as current and progressive—in each ego state, it follows that transactional analysis proper offers not only a theory of communication but also a powerful tool for thoroughly investigating the dynamics of transference and countertransference as well as authentic reciprocity, all of which underlie the relationships between human beings.

As communication tools, transactions constitute units of social exchange and were classified by Berne into complementary, crossed, and ulterior transactions. *Complementary transactions* establish symmetrical-type social relations whether healthy (i.e., directed toward mutual acknowledgment and support) or pathological (i.e., prone to symbiosis, dynamics of superiority-inferiority, or competitiveness). These are characterized in transactional diagrams with parallel vectors.

In contrast, crossed transactions are asymmetrical social exchanges that can again be separated into constructive and healthy (e.g., therapeutic operations aimed at disrupting dysfunctional intrapsychic processes and relational patterns) and pathological (e.g., those that may produce impairment or result in passivity and abrupt interruption of communication). These are characterized by crossed vectors.

Finally, *ulterior transactions*, which Berne classified into particular variants, occur not only outside the Adult's awareness but also travel along two levels of interchange: a social (or manifest) level and a psychological (or latent) level. As with other types of transaction, ulterior transactions may also result in constructive experiences for the individual (e.g., therapeutic paradoxes or therapies based on play) or can be destructive (e.g., the pathological *double bind* described by Weakland & Jackson as cited in Berne, 1975b [1961], p. 89, or in forms of manipulative relationships aimed at exploitation and social control). Unlike other transactions, ulterior transactions consist of two types of vectors that notably differentiate the social level (conscious) from the psychological level (preconscious and even unconscious) and can be parallel or crossed depending on the ego states involved in the transaction.

In one of his first works, "Concerning the nature of communication" (which appeared in *The Psychiatric Quarterly* in 1953; Berne 1977a [1953]), Berne explicitly referred to the importance of research carried out during those same years by Wiener (1948) on cybernetics. Berne followed with interest the then-new sensation that this discipline had started to create with its theoretical principles in diverse fields of knowledge, from mathematics to theoretical and applied physics and neurophysiology. He indicated how some physiologists, such as Ashby (1950) and Walter (1950, 1951), had used cybernetic systems to explain certain brain functions. It was precisely in echoing the cybernetic concepts of *information* and *noise*, carried over to psychology during those years by Ruesch and Bateson (1951), that Berne identified two levels of intrinsic messages in interpersonal communication: a manifest level (content) and a latent level (process or relationship), respectively. The argument about the nature of communication later came together in the Bernean idea of ulterior transaction, which is characterized by the duplex level—social and psychological—on which information (verbal and nonverbal) travels between two or more interlocutors.

Also, explicitly following the preliminary works of Weakland and Jackson on the same subject (Weakland & Jackson as cited in Berne, 1975b [1961], p. 89), Berne anticipated by around a decade the elaboration of certain of the most original ideas contained in the axioms of the later *Pragmatics of human communication* (Watzlawick et al., 1967) formulated by researchers from the Mental Research Institute in nearby Palo Alto, California. However, by that time transactional analysis had already been born and constituted not simply a theory of communication but also a much more comprehensive systematic and para-Freudian phenomenology with the ambitious aim of being able to provide "both clinically and theoretically ... a suitable context for the introduction of any other form of rational therapy" (Berne, 1977d [1966], p. 292).

On the other hand, a single transaction is a unique vehicle for thoughts, emotions, bodily experiences, and behavioral actions arising from past epochs as well as from current ego states in continual development. Particularly within psychotherapy, the various types of transaction are classified into two types: those analyst-patient relationships that involve transference and countertransference and those that are, instead, based on authenticity and intimacy (and therefore on mutual acknowledgment and growth) between two or more individuals. If we look closely at transactions—complementary, crossed, and ulterior—we can see that they are all susceptible to (not yet) conscious, preconscious, and even unconscious mental activity. This view was already implicit in Berne's transactional analysis concepts of transference and countertransference. It is worth noting how Berne's original focus limited the spectrum of his analytic exploration to intrapsychic and relational dynamics that are amenable to preconscious and conscious observation to the detriment of a larger unconscious phenomenology that also concerns the Adult ego state of the personality. Within the therapy room, in particular, transference and countertransference transactions, when they are integrated by the Adult—at first the Adult of the analyst and, in certain situations, also that of his or her supervisor—return to being at the service of the whole ego (the patient's as well as the analyst's) and can thereby bring about current trans-formative experiences. These are often inexpressible because they are still unconscious and (not yet) conscious cognitive, bodily-emotional, and beha-vioural experiences that feed into mutual interpersonal growth as result of the analytic process.

In this sense, transactional analysis also seems like a social psychology inasmuch as it proposes an actual theory of *among-ness*, that is, a being among others (seen here as a function of the integrating Adult) as well as being in relation to significant others from the person's past. This among-ness, a kind of middle ground between the self and the other, is what allows the unfolding of a bipersonal and multipersonal field of relationships that ulti-mately allows one's ego to disentangle defensive processes, loosen up its own rigidities, and achieve authentic reciprocity with other people.

In the beginning was "hello!"

In the opening lines of *What do you say after you say hello?*, Berne (1975c [1972]) indicated in laconic style how "to say 'hello' rightly is to see the other person, to be aware of him as a phenomenon, to happen to him and to be ready for him to happen to you" (p. 22). For Berne, becoming aware of the other as other-than-self means meeting that fundamental need—rooted in human biology and the experience of relating to peers (and in some cases even to certain animals)—to which he gave the name *recognition hunger*. The concept of hunger for Berne (1970, 1975c [1972]) retained the psychobiologi-cal and object relation qualities that were originally attributed in the psycho-analytic tradition to the concept of *desire* (or *tension*). In particular, the word *hunger* echoes simultaneously the concepts of *drive* (rooted in the body with its polarities of libido and mortido), which is central to the (neo-)Freudian model of the psyche, and *need* (with its relational modalities of love and hate), which is more in tune with a post-Freudian relational view of the psy-chodynamic stream.

Recognition hunger is also viewed as being socially derived from—and in a certain sense sublimated to—*sensation hunger*, the vital need for actual sensory stimulation of an interbodily kind (including physical contact) as experienced by human beings from the earliest phases of perinatal and neonatal life:

> Most people have a hunger for human contact, at least of sight and sound, and in most cases also for touch or stroking. ... Such contact may actually make the difference between physical and mental health or breakdown, and even between life and death.
>
> (Berne, 1970, p. 190)

Transactional analysis theory, unlike the Freudian psychoanalytic model, distinguishes within the original *hunger for Other* the subject's primary need for human relationships. Berne (1977d [1966]) defined the unit of mutual recognition as a "'stroke,' by analogy to physical caressing in infancy" (p. 230). It is fascinating to note that, because the transaction is a unit of social exchange, each transaction inevitably involves an exchange of strokes. There are two large conceptual references clearly at work at this point in Berne's explanation. They concern the basic function of the relationship with the other for the individual's healthy psychophysical development. On the one hand, there are the pioneering clinical trials conducted by Rene Spitz (1945) on institutionalized children deprived of or lacking consistent maternal presence and care. On the other, there are the important contributions to the ethological field in the studies of Harlow and Harlow (1962) on social deprivation in rhesus monkeys, the studies of sensory stimulation in mice by Levine (1960) (as cited in Berne 1977d [1966], p. 260), and Lorenz's discoveries (1952) on imprinting in ducks (as cited in Berne, 1970, p. 113).

In fact, Berne, with his subsequent emphasis on the *typology of strokes* (positive/negative, conditional/unconditional)—designed as units of syntonic (or, in contrast, dystonic) mutual recognition between individuals engaged in a transaction—implicitly introduced a kind of bidirectional progression to his transactional analysis model of the mind and human relationships. In other words, it is possible to find in the Bernean role of recognition hunger and hunger for strokes a powerful anticipation of what will be the relational (i.e., bipersonal) turning point in psychoanalytic theory.

Moreover, Berne (1975c [1972]) also observed how, for recognition by the other in his or her role as other-than-self to happen, it is first necessary to "see" the other person. This means, from a bipersonal perspective, to be greeted "correctly" by the other, which means to be seen by the other and consequently received by the other unconditionally. The decisive importance of the other's attention—including the original reference other (i.e., the Other)—for maintaining our sense of identity and health throughout life is encapsulated well in this somewhat provocative extract from Berne:

As the individual grows up, he learns to accept symbolic forms of stroking instead of the actual touch, until the mere act of recognition serves the purpose. ... What is said is less important than the fact that people are recognizing each other's presence and in that way offering the social contact which is necessary for the preservation of health. Thus both infants and grownups show a need for, or at least an appreciation of, social contact even in its most primitive forms. This can be easily tested by anyone who has the courage to refuse to respond when his friends say "Hello."

(Berne, 1975a [1963], p. 215)

Berne assigned strokes—which act as a bridge between the intrapsychic and relational worlds—a central role in the healthy psychophysical development of the individual as well as for the transformative processes supported by analytic therapy. Similarly, those strokes that result in a lack of recognition or dystonic recognition (i.e., distorted, significantly early, or delayed in time) are believed to be responsible for *developmental disharmony* (to use an expression from Anna Freud (1965), another reference author for Berne) and therefore for subsequent psychopathological deviations from development. These are thought to be as serious as the failure to meet the hunger for strokes, a failure that is early and enduring.

From this perspective, it follows that all those microenvironmental events that have somehow ignored, denied, or even threatened the satisfaction of the individual's recognition hunger, and that are characterized as real transactional experiences with significant others from the person's past, make up actual *relational traumas* that can accumulate like a "pile of coins" (Berne, 1975b [1961], p. 53) and lie more or less stratified, decomposed, and even fragmented in the psyche. This does not mean that fantasy life carried any less weight for Berne in terms of generating psychopathological symptoms. Rather, the contribution made by the person's real experiences, particularly if they are traumatic, can be etched to a large degree on their (pre)conscious as well as unconscious (not necessarily repressed) activity. They thereby interact throughout life with neurodevelopmental processes that are the basis for different kinds of memory, attention, schema and bodily images, imagination (including dream activity), and spoken language, just to mention the most important few.

Ascribing to relational trauma—especially if it is multifaceted and cumulative—the structural origin (i.e., historical and progressive) of psychopathology, Berne initially made use of Breuer and Freud's (1955 [1895]) thesis concerning the emotional-traumatic genesis of psychic disorders. This suggested that the psychopathological symptom (in specific cases such as hysteria) was brought back to the level of the patient's relationships and of the traumatic events (almost invariably sexual) that had marked the person's life story (Freud, 1955a [1917]). This prepsychoanalytic view of psychopathology—which Berne fundamentally reframed with his multipartite view of the mind in terms of discrete ego states—is implicitly connected to Janet's (1889, 1908) *analyse psychologique*, which, in turn, related psychopathological experiences that tend to be inherent in the human psyche to structural *dissociation*, understood as the main psychological process through which the individual reacts to a traumatic event.

It is worth mentioning that this theoretical position in 1956—appearing exactly at the time Berne (1977e [1949], 1977b [1952], 1977c [1955]) was working on intuition and the phenomenology of the ego—meant that his application for the title of psychoanalyst from the San Francisco Psychoanalytic Institute was refused. It is interesting to note what John Bowlby (1988), whose attachment theory led him to distance himself (albeit with less impetus than Berne) from psychoanalysis based on a model of the mind mainly driven by impulses, wrote some decades later:

> That was a time when Freud's famous about-turn of 1897 regarding the aetiology of hysteria had led to the view that anyone who places emphasis on what a child's real experiences may have been, and perhaps still are being, was regarded as pitifully naïve.
>
> (p. 43)

For Berne, in fact, it was precisely this refusal to grant him entry into the psychoanalytic establishment at that time that steered him toward full reappropriation of the theory of relational trauma he had postulated as the foundation of a new transactional analytic psychology:

> Structural analysis is concerned with … the relics of the infant who once actually existed, in a struggle with the relics of the parents who once actually existed. The struggle is described here in anthropomorphic terms just because it retains its personal quality: it is not a battle between abstract conceptualized forces, but reduplicates the actual childhood fights for survival between real people, or at least that is the way the patient experiences it.
>
> (Berne, 1975b [1961], p. 66)

Within this perspective, it is precisely relational trauma—resulting in a fight for survival—that is deemed the pathogenetic factor in processes of intrapsychic conflict and structural deficit with which psychopathology in a psychodynamic sense is classically defined and that find in Berne's concepts of *contamination* and *exclusion* a powerful theoretical illustration that is still valid today.

Pathology of Ego Boundaries

The transactional dimension of the ego, with its psychopathological and healthy variations, is based on the hypothesis that internal and external boundaries exist to a particular relationship between two or more people. Staying in the clinical setting, internal boundaries to the analytic relationship are principally intraegoic boundaries (i.e., those between the various ego states of individuals) and interegoic boundaries (i.e., those between ego states belonging to two or more people involved in the same relationship). External boundaries, on the other hand, are those of the analytic setting itself and more generally of everything that separates the analytic from the extra-analytic dimension (e.g., the physical walls of the therapy room, the timetable and frequency of the sessions, the type of therapy contract, etc.).

Berne's transactional analysis theory recognized the structural genesis of psychopathological symptoms of the personality in the intrapsychic processes of contamination and exclusion, which can be translated as significant alterations in intraegoic and interegoic boundaries (Berne, 1975b [1961], pp. 44–51).

In other words, contamination and exclusion for Berne are structural macro-organizations that the ego uses to deal with traumatic relational situations along the individual's entire psychodevelopmental course. As such, contamination and exclusion bring together a large number of adaptation processes—better known in psychoanalysis as *defense mechanisms*—which, on the one hand, are proof of the service of internal organization provided by these to their ego and, on the other hand, indicate the places understood together as intrapsychic and relational *topoi* (from the Greek *topos* meaning "place" and similarly "type"), where the psychopathological distortions of an individual reside.

Contamination was described by Berne (1975b [1961], pp. 47–50) as the nonconscious intrusion of a part of one or more ego states into another ego state. Nonconscious intrusion means that the ego state involved in the process of contamination—be it the Parent, the Adult, and/or the Child—perceives the experiences from other contaminating ego systems as syntonic with its own ego system. For example, if the Adult ego state is actively involved in the contamination process, it follows that intrusive experiences coming from the Parent (e.g., in the form of prejudices), from the Child (e.g., in the form of hallucinatory phenomena), or both (double contamination) are included in the ego organization of the Adult and exchanged for facts of reality.

Contamination, at least as Berne thought of it, reflects a vision of psychopathology based on intrapsychic conflict but, once again, within a clear Freudian prepsychoanalytic and para-Freudian matrix. Berne's view, in contrast to Freud's intrapsychic impulse model, undoubtedly considered the conflict dimension to be implicit in relationality. In this he was in line with the object dimension of conflict originally propounded by Melanie Klein (1952):

The analysis of very young children has taught me that there is no instinctual urge, no anxiety situation, no mental process that does not involve objects, external or internal; in other words, object-relations are at the centre of emotional life. Furthermore, love and hatred,

12

phantasies, anxieties, and defences are also operative from the beginning and are *ab initio* indivisibly linked with object-relations.

(p. 434)

In contrast to structural models of conflict that postulate the existence of predetermined ego drives and organizations—and in part this was also Klein's supposition—transactional analysis understands intrapsychic conflict as an anthropomorphic precipitate of relational conflicts that actually existed and are still ongoing at the psychological level for the individual. Intrapsychic conflict is, therefore, the result of an internalization of conflicting relationships with significant others. In this way, Berne's theory of ego states continues to have more in common with object relation theorists such as Fairbairn, Guntrip, and even Winnicott than with Freud's and, to some extent, Klein's psychoanalysis (Bateman, Brown, & Pedder, 2009 [1979], pp. 46–47).

Moreover, Berne's thesis on contamination as a dynamic process that imbues the ego in different phases of its development and organization is in complete agreement with the epigenetic theory of his analyst Erik Erikson (1993 [1950], 1963), who specifically identified a series of epigenetic stages throughout life characterized by distinct psychosocial crises. In this way, Erikson's view, unlike that of Freud and Klein, extends his developmental theory beyond childhood and adolescence. Further, Erikson argued that for each psychodevelopmental stage, the existence of a conflict is not primarily between drives within the subject but rather of a psychosocial, relational nature. For each psychosocial crisis, the individual is not primarily faced with endopsychic impulses to satisfy and a struggle with the demands of society but with a series of existential tasks to be solved within the network of relationships in which the person is included.

In the foregoing considerations one can see how the transactional analysis theory of the personality undoubtedly considers and expands, through Berne's teaching on contamination, the conflict dimension of existence. This dimension is understood in terms of a conflict that is both intrapsychic and relational, where the protagonists in the struggle are ego states or anthropomorphic precipitates of affective, bodily, cognitive, and behavioral experiences that have all inevitably emerged and are emerging within significant relationships.

Given the plural nature of the ego as proposed by Berne (1975b [1961]), exclusion refers to one or more pathological discontinuities within the personality structure of the individual. Such ego fractures—classically diagrammed by Berne (1975b [1961]) as dashed circles (see Figure 1.2)—identify intrapsychic voids, that is, anthropomorphic precipitates of historical relational deficiencies (and/or divides) and even nonrelationship between the developing individual and his or her reference others. These excluded parts of the personality are, counterintuitively, "active absences" of the Other(s) in that they might be able to function as "black holes" at different stages of psychodevelopment, both intrapsychically and relationally, by preventing more corrective identifications of the self with a new potentially regulatory other(s). This could ultimately undermine the development within the self (via internalization) of a more three-dimensional (i.e., psychological, relational, and bodily) sense of the Other(s) and even compromise the perception of the other(s) as other(s)-than-self. It is this process that is said to be operating, for example, during psychotic states of mind.

Because no human being can actually survive in a world of adults with a completely excluded Adult, it follows that exclusion usually involves the Parent or Child ego state with an Adult that is more or less sufficiently developed and integrated (Figure 1.2). The ego state that is particularly active in the process of exclusion, acting *inter alia* as almost the only regulator of intraego and transactional dynamics, was identified by Berne as the *excluding* ego state. This ego state is excluding because of the thickening of its ego boundaries and therefore its structural rigidity, which is then expressed at the phenomenological level as a series of stereotyped, sustained, predictable, and often "frozen" manifestations of the person's personality (Berne, 1975b [1961], pp. 44–47, 51).

In this regard, Berne emphasized the adaptive and defensive function of the exclusion process when he wrote this:

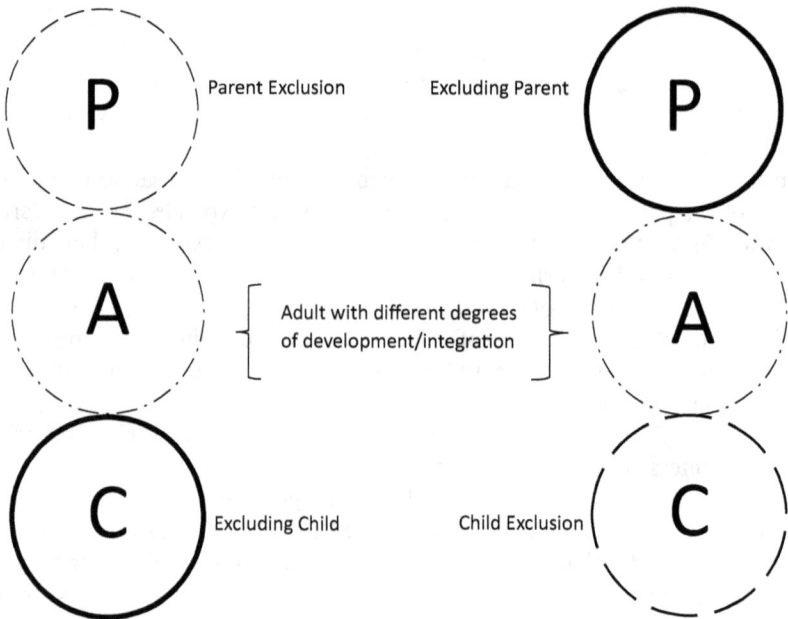

Figure 1.2 Exclusion(s) (adapted from Berne, 1975b [1961], p.46)

The clinical problem presented by such pathological exclusions demonstrates both the function and the nature of the paramount ego state. Attempts to communicate with the excluded aspects are frustrated by the idiosyncratic response of the defending Parent, Adult, or Child.

(Berne, 1975b [1961], p. 47)

In other words, the concept of the excluding ego state enabled Berne to identify another process capable of generating psychopathology: the developmental arrest of the ego in specific areas—corresponding to definite psychodevelopmental periods—of its current structural organization. Exclusion, as proposed by Berne in his ego state model, fully reflects the conceptual paradigm of the structural deficit in psychopathology, according to which mental suffering originates in a complex system of defenses and adaptations put in place to overcome traumatic relational deficiencies experienced by the individual during specific phases of psychophysical development.

Specifically, Berne echoed, and to some extent anticipated, the constitutive function of relational deficit in generating psychopathology as pioneered by two leading figures in clinical psychoanalysis at the time: Helene Deutsch and Anna Freud. In particular, Deutsch—whom Berne (1975b [1961]) described as "a thoughtful psychoanalyst of wide experience" (p. 261)—introduced the concept of the *as-if* in her article from 1942 entitled "Some forms of emotional disturbance and their relationship to schizophrenia." In it she described how the origin of some forms of psychopathology can be traced back to a preconflictual or even an a-conflictual dimension of psychodevelopment in which "relationships devoid of any trace of warmth," an "atmosphere lacking in feelings," and an "affective deficiency" (p. 303) may be created in the relationship between infant and primary caregiving figures. This argument was, to some extent, reprised by Anna Freud (1965), who, in *Normality and pathology in childhood: Assessments of development*, described two types of childhood psychopathology: one that is conflict based and the other which is grounded in psychodevelopmental arrests deriving from a highly dysfunctional environment (including family life).

Berne seems to have anticipated Winnicott with a theory, in part derived from studies of Deutsch's work, according to which the most archaic experiential layers attributable to the Child ego state may occur and stratify in the psyche early in life. Specifically, these are unlanguaged experiences of mutuality that are phenomenologically (re)expressed—far beyond childhood and throughout development—according to and in an as-if modality as represented through the concepts of Adapted Child and Natural Child (Berne, 1975b [1961]). Like the Winnicottian "True Self" and "False Self" (Winnicott, 1965, pp. 140–152), the nature of the Child ego state, in both its Adapted and Natural modalities, is conceivable in that it is intrinsically related to the Parent. As such it coincides with the internalization of the

15

relational dynamics between the developing infant and primary parental (or alloparental) figures. In Berne's (1975b [1961]) own words, "The adapted Child is an archaic ego state which is under the Parental influence, while the natural Child is an archaic ego state which is free from or is attempting to free itself from such influence" (p. 42).

Boundaries of psychopathology (and mental health)

Given the relational nature of ego states, every pathology borne by intraego boundaries corresponds with an alteration in interego boundaries, with the result that intrapsychic pathos is contextually a suffering "in the presence of" the Other, making the Other suffer, suffering with the Other. Translated into more clinical terms, having a mental disorder—even in those conditions of almost ineffable suffering—invariably means being in a real predicament, that is, in a situation in which the individual comes to live, relive, and hopefully find relief from past and current struggles and frustrations in the relationship with more or less significant others (including the analyst).

The mental suffering that the individual experiences idiosyncratically and endogenously retains an intersubjective dimension of a notably historical-relational and, at the same time, progressive nature that needs to be somehow revealed and transformed within the actual analytic relationship. In other words, the transference that patients actualize within the psychotherapeutic relationship serves two main, and usually unconscious, purposes. On the one hand, it makes the person's past relationships phenomenologically available to the therapist's scrutiny and his or her protective containment; on the other, it demands the transformative presence of and engagement with a new trusting other who will actively allow the patient to keep developing and therefore to progress on his or her own personal journey.

At this point there can be no progress in the transactional analytic investigation of the (inter)subjective experience of mental suffering conducted thus far without a consideration of the Other. So who is this Other that transactional analysis will deal with?

The Other is primarily the Parent (Figure 1.3), understood as the (pre)ego internalization of the relationship with the original parent from the perinatal and infantile period (P_0, P_1). It is also the parent and any other figure in *loco parentis* who stands out, starting from the second infancy (around 2–6 years) and childhood (around 7–12 years) onward, against the internal background of our subjectivity as both regulatory and emotional authority (P_2, P_2, P_n, or $P_{umpteenth}$).

The Other is also the therapist who can become a new Other or new Parent (P_0, P_1, P_2, P_3, P_n) for the patient. The Other is the then, the now, and the not-yet: it carries with it the memory of the past, the signs and signals of wounds and relational deficits that are still present, and the first signs of healing, growth, and hope for the future. The Other is, potentially, the not-yet-present as well as the

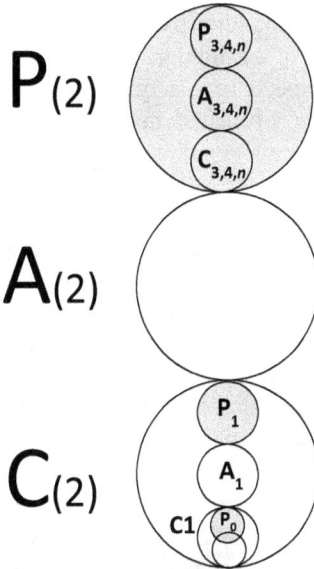

Figure 1.3 The Parent ego state from a developmental perspective (adapted from Berne, 1975b [1961], p. 193)

great-absent, the unknown, and the mysterious. Even more generally, the Other is simultaneously the ubiquitous and the oblique, meaning, respectively, with the former, the potential ubiquitousness of the Other because of transferential processes (including projective-introjective identifications), and with the latter, the asymmetry of its transactions (such as crossed and ulterior transactions) on which depend processes of developmental arrest as well as processes of growth and individuation of the self.

Ultimately, the Other as *transactional subject* is what makes possible and real both internal among-ness (ego states) and interpersonal among-ness (states in transaction between real people). The problem of the self in relation to the Other can be resolved within this basic condition of human subjectivity, which is precisely that of "existing among" both inside and outside of ourselves.

This existing among is a middle ground, a continuous becoming from which subjectivity and otherness can emerge. For Berne (1975b [1961]), the ultimate attempt of humans to inhabit this middle ground becomes an actual *life script*, that is, "a whole transference drama, often split up into acts, exactly like the theatrical scripts which are intuitive artistic derivatives of these primal dramas of childhood" (p. 116).

Following on from Freud—and more so from the main works of such successors as Otto Rank (2015 [1909]), Carl Jung (2016 [1921]), and Alfred Adler

(2011 [1924])—life script is the term that Berne (1975c [1972], Chapter 3) gave to the existential dramas of all human beings, that is, the reason why their needs, aspirations, and expectations acquire an early and enduring (lifelong) mobility and why their ways of satisfying and realizing them are constructed in such a way as to form an experiential plan and destiny. In this regard, Berne (1975c [1972]) clarified how "of all those who preceded transactional analysis, Alfred Adler comes the closest to talking like a script analyst" (p. 80), relating the Adlerian idea of an *unconscious life plan* ("secret life plan") with the life script, as Berne called it.

Following a kind of phenomenological heuristic in this way, Berne revisited the Freudian interpretation of the myth of Oedipus: "In psychoanalytic language ... Oedipus is something going on in the patient's head. In script analysis, Oedipus is an ongoing drama that is actually taking place right now, divided into scenes and acts, with a build-up, a climax, and an ending" (Berne, 1975c [1972], p. 79). This is, in my view, the most radical step taken by Berne on the theme of the Oedipus complex. Oedipus is not a cornerstone of transactional analysis but a myth among many existing myths, legends, and fairy tales with which one can reread the existence of the single individual from an essentially sociological and collective perspective. It is no coincidence that Berne's text makes explicit reference to Joseph Campbell (2008 [1949]), whose work *The hero with a thousand faces* was singled out by Berne (1975c [1972]) as "the best textbook for script analysts" (p. 68).

Ultimately, developing a life script means for Berne's tragic human being to essentially try and answer existential questions such as "Who am I?" "Who is the other?" "What am I to the other?" "What is the other to me?" "Where do we come from?" "Where are we going?" "What may happen to someone like me?" "What does this world, nature, mean to us?" But inasmuch as it is a repetitive scenario that belongs to the phenomenon of transference, the script is, for Berne (1977d [1966], p. 368), an unconscious life plan that may nevertheless emerge at a preconscious and unconscious level of experience inherent in the analytic experience. The parts that comprise the script are not mere roles but the personification of unconscious and preconscious ego states, and therefore the reactualization of relational experiences related to different eras of the person's psychological development. In the same way that a theatrical script (play) consists of acts, and acts are made up of scenes and scenes of lines, similarly the script drama unfolds in *games*.

In particular, the psychological games about which Berne (1975b [1961], Chapter 10; 2008 [1964]; 1977d [1966], Chapter 14; 1970, Chapter 5; 1975c [1972], Chapters 2, 8) wrote are basically dysfunctional relational patterns that are established over time but still repeatedly "staged" in the present at a conscious (first-degree games) or mostly preconscious and even unconscious level of expression (second- and third-degree games).

The theory of psychological games is also a very Bernean reinterpretation—based on a direct observational as well as analytic method—of Freud's

(1955b [1920]) *compulsion to repeat*. In Berne's view, the game draws its vitality from an often unfavorable emotional *payoff* for the individuals in the same way that the life script is seen as moving toward a usually tragic finale. On this conceptual cohesion between psychological games and script, Berne essentially never wavered. This is indeed a sensitive point in Berne's thinking in which Bateson's lecture on paradoxical communications—which was referred to regarding ulterior transactions—is again particularly trenchant (Bateson, 1956 as cited in Berne, 1975b [1961], pp. 88–89) but with a precise cultural leap to the work *Homo ludens* by Danish historian Johan Huizinga (2016 [1938]). With the transactional analysis theory of psychological games, Berne radicalized in an original way the position of Huizinga on the intimate relationship between games and civilization. For Berne, the social dimension of human existence in all its emotionally salient manifestations—with the sole exception of true intimacy—finds expression and actualization *sub specie ludi*. Because the essential feature of human play lies in the fact that in play there are (even authentic) emotions subjected to rules (Cornell, 2015a), *psychological games*, which Berne's transactional analysis deals with, in particular, can be anything but banally "playful"; on the contrary, they risk being a "deadly serious, or even fatally serious" affair (Berne, 1975b [1961], p. 88).

The bipersonal (if not even polypersonal) nature of the psychological game is not as evident in Berne's original theory formulation as it is in the work of subsequent authors in the transactional analytic field, such as Cornell (2015a, 2016), Hine (1990), Novak (2015), Stuthridge (2015), and Stuthridge and Sills (2016). Nevertheless, the transactional analysis value placed on psychological games by Berne remains unchanged. This value is duplex. On the one hand, games are rather complex adaptive (including defensive) relational patterns linked to frustrations and early relational traumas experienced by the person in his or her original family (not necessarily biological), traumas that are at risk of (re-)presenting in the here and now. On the other, games have an informative quality; they offer, especially in the analytic setting via transference and countertransference dynamics, direct and co-lived access to the not-immediately conscious and unconscious intrapsychic and relational world of the individual. In other words, games are a phenomenological means to enter a person's actual life script and even protocol experiences.

At a deeper level of reflection, the *conditio sine qua non* for the structuring of a life script and its preconscious and conscious components is, in Berne's view, the assumption of a basic *life position*. The life position allows the emerging ego to give an object position (and therefore a relational position) and a sense of value to one's own self, to the other, and to life in general. For this reason, a life position, according to Berne (1977d [1966], pp. 270–271; 1975c [1972], pp. 110–120), is the expression of a bipersonal I-You and multipersonal I-You-others relationship. The ideal or healthy life position was identified by Berne (1975c [1972], pp. 111–112) as "I'm OK, You're OK." Against this are counterposed the contrasting positions: "I'm OK, You're not

OK" (paranoia), "I'm not OK, You're OK" (depression), and "I'm not OK, You're not OK" (schizoid).

This essential chapter of Berne's theory clearly follows Melanie Klein's (1997a [1957], 1997b [1952], 1997c [1932]) point of view on positions—schizoid-paranoid and depressive—assumed by the infant from the first year of life. Berne not only borrowed the terminology from Klein but explicitly acknowledged its cultural legacy (Berne, 1977d [1966]). However, Klein's positions underwent a temporal extension in Berne, one that goes beyond the infant period to potentially characterize an individual's entire existence to the point where, as Berne (1977d [1966]) wrote, "every game, script and destiny is based on one of these four basic positions" (p. 270). In substance, this is a temporal as well as substantial development of Klein's theory on positions. In other words, Klein's positions become basic positions in Berne (1977d [1966]), that is, relational positions (I-You) underpinning the individual's existence and characterizing his or her relationship patterns into adulthood and beyond. If the reader asked for a conceptual comparison to explain the heuristic significance of Berne's thesis on basic positions, one could say that these have the same value in the transactional analytic field as the concepts of *secure base* and *attachment styles* assumed in the work of John Bowlby and his later developments in psychotherapy.

Everything that happens before the individual assumes a more conscious existential I-You position is related to the ineffable and early neonatal (even intrauterine) and infant period of life, during which nonverbal, preverbal, and unconscious relationship experiences are formed between the individual and primary caregiving figures. These experiences find a nonconscious narrative through affectively shaped bodies, even before a differentiated I and You are established in the individual's consciousness. Berne (1975b [1961], 1977d [1966], 1975c [1972]) called this *protocol*. As the internalization of the earliest unconscious patterns of the person's relationship with significant others, the protocol is considered to be a crude and preliminary version of the later life script, the latter understood as transferential drama, the origin of which, as mentioned earlier, is notably located in the earliest infant period.

The protocol is also conceived in this book as one of the clinical keys that opens the way to understanding and treating the schizophrenic experience from a transactional analysis perspective. However, given the small and fairly patchy discussion by Berne on this topic, I have, of necessity, turned to works produced by other authoritative figures in transactional analysis on the formation of script and therefore the nature of protocol (Caizzi, 2012; Cornell, 2005, 2010, 2015b; Cornell & Landaiche, 2006, 2008; Guglielmotti, 2008; Ligabue, 2007; Pierini, 2008). Personal experience gained through years of clinical work with schizophrenic patients, many of them experiencing their first psychotic episode, has led me to believe, along with the aforementioned authors, that the protocol is a transactional area of our psychic life and relationships with high emotional charge and with influences that extend far beyond early childhood to affect the whole of our existence. Specifically, pro-tocol—fundamentally understood as the *tissue level* of existence (Berne, 1975c [1972])—corresponds with a wider and always active sensed, polysensory, interbodily, nonconscious, and nonverbal dimension of the human experience of being and being in relation to someone. It is, in other words, a fluid and creative dimension of being where the I and the You, the self and the other, have not (yet) found mutual differentiation.

Since Berne's suggestive writing in this area, this interbodily, tissue level of the experience of relating has found broad resonance in the psychoanalytic literature (Mahler, Pine, & Bergman 1975; Stern 1985, 1990, 1995), including, more recently, in the clinical work and research of contemporary psycho-analysts and psychotherapists such Bollas (1987, 1989), Bucci (1997, 2008), and Cornell (2015b).

Psychopathology, according to Berne, transcends the intrapsychic to result in repeated, and not always updated, editions of (inter)ego (life positions, rackets, games, script) and even pre-ego or not-yet ego (protocol) transac-tional experiences that occur outside Adult awareness. And all that together belongs to the unconscious (not necessarily repressed) realm of the psyche and therefore as much to processes of transference as countertransference, especially when these are (re)lived in the analytic arena. By contrast, mental health is not necessarily the opposite of script, understood here as the con-tinuous daily texture of our lives. Rather, we are given a particular intrap-sychic and relational life precisely because of the search for a continuous adaptation to reality, adaptation that finds in the protocol, in its subsequent adolescent revisioning, and ultimately in the continual development of the life script the expression of a creative *poiesis* of the self in its attempts to adapt to, while often defending itself from and even endeavoring to escape from, the traumatic relationship with the Other.

From this perspective, mental health—as well as the transactional analytic treatment to facilitate and promote it—achieves a coherence, in Berne's view, with a much broader human condition than the mere absence of psycho-pathology. It becomes, instead, an ethical act, namely, an act of personal responsibility toward the self, the other, and life in general.

Preparing for intimacy

Since the ego is not even master in its own house (Freud, 1955a [1917])—but, as ego, finds itself inhabited by a multitude of ego state entities, first among which is the Other as Parent —the individual is precluded once and for all from any possibility of true autonomy. Autonomy, in the strictest sense, is an illusion, and Berne (1970, p. 178) stated this mercilessly at times. The natural condition of human existence is, instead, that of *heteronomy* (from the Greek *heteros* meaning "other as different" and *nomos* meaning "law"), understood as regarding the law of the Other, of that which is different from us. And the law of the Other is not the same for everyone. There is never, nor can there ever be, a Parent that is the same as another, not even when it is one's own biological parent. Thus, the person cannot follow a personal, and therefore autonomous, law (from the Greek *autos* meaning "own" and *nomos* meaning "law") that does not take into account the ever-present relationship with the others. It is in this paradoxical, altruistic exercise of autonomy that the individual can (re)encounter the other and therefore his or her own self with awareness, spontaneity, and intimacy (Berne, 2008 [1964], Chapter 16; 1977d [1966], pp. 306–307; 1970, p. 105, pp. 125–130).

Moreover, the problem of the self—of a self that is never complete—rests on the same philosophical foundations. In fact, becoming oneself is a process of actualization in constant evolution of one's own ego in transaction with the other. This constant evolution is irredeemably linked to the passing of time and to how it is structured by the person according to a level of growing transactional involvement: from isolation to rituals, pastimes, activities, psychological games, and intimacy (Berne, 2008 [1964], pp. 15–19). On this scale, which puts intimacy at the pinnacle—or, if you like, at the foundation—of more compelling and unsettling transactional experiences for the human being, the individual experiences different degrees of ontological uncertainty and insecurity. That is why the way the individual structures his or her waking hours is both an expression of his or her degree of health (as well as mental suffering) and an eminently existential problem.

Indeed, from an existential and existentialistic perspective dear to Bernean thinking—as demonstrated by Berne's many references to philosophers such as Kierkegaard and Sartre (Berne, 1975a [1963], pp. 156, 232; 2008 [1964], p. 17; 1977d [1966], pp. 278, 316; 1975b [1961], p. 89)—the subject is somehow able to pass through time rather than to see it simply slide past in the hands of a clock (Berne, 1970, p. 210). The individual's time is, in other words, a time that is always and irredeemably lived and whose way of being structured in conditions of psychopathology alternates between two extremes: on the one hand, personal isolation, which leads to withdrawal and estrangement from the world of relationships, and on the other, *confusion*, which substitutes for healthy reciprocity based on a mutual recognition. The former (i.e., isolation) indicates the traumatic lack of the Other; the latter (i.e., con-fusion) the phagocytosis—sometimes observable in psychological games—of the Other. Both these extremes—isolation and confusion—retain, however, irreducible cores of potential health and interpersonal growth: solitude and intimacy, respectively. This alternation of lived time echoes certain reflections by Kierkegaard on boredom, reflections that Berne (1975b [1961], pp. 88–89) emphasized when he placed the existential problem of boredom at the center of his transactional analysis theory of the social relationship. The Kierkegaardian boredom mentioned by Berne—and that Berne's person seeks to overcome through the structuring of time—does not lead inexorably to the petrification of existence but is, rather—as, indeed, is the ego—a "condensation of possibility" (Kierke-gaard, 1991 [1845], p. 428), a life in a constant paradox, a "superficial pro-fundity" and a "hungry satiety" (Kierkegaard, 1968 [1841], p. 302).

Put another way, the time of subjectivity is also the time to live (or not) one's own freedom, or at least to follow the desire to do so. But, as we have seen, subjective time is a time defined by the Other. If, in order to be free, the person must stop and think and, an even more arduous task, give up the illusion of autonomy, to achieve singularity (i.e., to be unique and unrepea-table), he or she needs solitude *and* intimacy. The person needs to treat himself or herself as an other-than-self and the other as himself or herself. The first is an *ethical* act—expressing a "moral responsibility" of the ego toward itself (or part of itself)—and the second is an act of *pathos*, that is, an exercise that is responsible for emotional receptivity toward the new other (Berne, 1975b [1961], pp. 193–195). From this it follows that even mental health, as the exercise of a law shared with the other, is fundamen-tally family, social, organizational, and even "political" health (from the Greek *polis* for "city" or "community"), with profound implications for an entire community (large or small) of individuals.

On the basis of these considerations, it is clear how Berne's transactional analysis theory of personality and human relationships corresponds with a philanthropic view, which finds its highest expression precisely in the uncon-ditional respect for the uniqueness of the other and in an authentic reciprocity (OK-ness). In clinical practice, this is reflected in a similarly philanthropic attitude by the therapist:

> [When preparing to meet with the patient] psychologically ... the therapist clears his mind of everything that has gone before in the way of preparation, of all that he knows about the patients, of all his personal problems, and of everything he has learned about psychiatry and psychotherapy. At his best, he becomes like an innocent new-born babe who has passed under the arch of his office doorway into a world he never made.
>
> (Berne, 1977d [1966], p. 62)

When they finally find themselves immersed in the particular context of the analytic relationship, a relationship different from any other, the Bernean analyst, whether working in an individual or group setting, is required to be essentially a humanistic psychotherapist. He or she must be able to make his or her own the Hippocratic foundations of the human sciences espoused in *primum non nocere* and *vis medicatrix naturae* (Berne, 1977d [1966], pp. 62–63) or *physis* (Berne, 1969 [1957], pp. 369–370); focus on recognizing the intrinsic worth of every individual and his or her autonomous ambitions (Berne, 1975c [1972], pp. 157–158); center on the here and now of the rela-tionship with the other; be aware of the current presence of the past and the transformative power of present relationships; be an attentive participant of transferential and countertransferential (and also interbodily) processes within the therapeutic encounter; and be an advocate, via the contract, for joint responsibility between patient and analyst in the therapeutic process.

These are the salient aspects of transactional analytic work in the clinical arena, particularly at a historical and economic-political time when the identity processes of many are wavering because the fundamental pillars of mental health are being threatened, including romantic relationships and work as well as personal and community safety. With the context of socioemotional and political insecurity in which we currently find ourselves, the analytic session becomes an even more valuable meeting place between two or more people. This is also why using a therapeutic contract becomes an additional tool in the protection of the suffering and freedom of individuals. The contract is also the fulcrum around which more or less effective, and especially ethical, techniques and methodologies for treatment are based insofar as they promote and/or give back power, permissions, and protection to the patient-individual within a relationship of authentic reciprocity as well as psychological and interpersonal growth.

Prolegomena to the transactional analysis of schizophrenic psychoses

The transactional analysis approach to schizophrenia discussed in this book concerns direct clinical practice with adult patients, including those experiencing prodromal signs of a psychotic breakdown, first episode schizophrenic patients, and those who are chronic but considered to be relapsing into an acute phase of their mental disorder. All the ideas and views, coming not only from the field of transactional analysis but also from the most relevant psychoanalytic contributions and recent advances, as well as experts' opinions on neuroscientific research in this field, share a common set of basic assumptions.

Neuroscientific research has generated as much evidence as controversy about the nature of schizophrenia

The idea that schizophrenic patients might experience a progressive decline in their mental, physical, and social abilities was supported by initial psychiatric speculations on the nature and course of this mental disorder, often coupled with longitudinal observations of patients in highly institutionalized settings.

Similarly, in the field of neuroscientific research, two main hypotheses about the pathophysiology of schizophrenia have attracted considerable attention over the years in the worldwide community of neuroscientists: the neurodegenerative and the neurodevelopmental models. The first stems from a Kraepelinian view of schizophrenia as a single disease (i.e., *dementia praecox*) by placing an intrinsically progressive neurodegenerative process at the core of schizophrenic pathology; the second is in line with a more Bleulerian view of schizophrenia as a "fragmented mind" thought to be embracing a clinically heterogeneous and mixed group of etiologically neurodevelopmentally derived syndromes.

Researchers in the field of biological psychiatry have held both of these views dichotomously or complementarily. However, it is my opinion that both of these neurobiological hypotheses, even when integrated into a unitary, twofold model, failed to acknowledge the iatrogenic impact of psychotropic medications on brain changes and thereby distorted clinicians' perspectives on phenomenological aspects and prognosis of this psychiatric syndrome. Moreover, these two models, even many years after their original formulation, did not comprehensively explore the more subtle interactions between biological and environmental (early biological insults, use of illicit drugs, etc.) as well as social factors (including traumatic childhood experiences, severe mental illness of caregivers, etc.) that are contributing factors to the development of schizophrenia. These complex interactions have, instead, become the focus of more recent research models that have combined evidence from brain pathology, structural and functional neuroimaging, gene-environment studies, epidemiology, neuropsychology, and social and psychological factors.

Symbiosis is an insufficient paradigm for understanding schizophrenic experiences

In healthy development, as infants we all become naturally symbiotic with our caregivers, which means that symbiosis necessarily has a healthy adaptive function. However, when applied to schizophrenic pathology, symbiosis, both in transactional analysis and the wider psychoanalytic literature, often refers not to an adaptive process but to a more fundamental regression of the ego to the earliest stages of psychodevelopment. Such a regression of the ego was originally thought to be a condition showing resistance and even no susceptibility to analytic treatment. Therefore, the term *symbiosis* tends to be misleading because it does not capture the progressive, rather than regressive, quality of psychotic processes implicated in active schizophrenia.

I would, instead, use the term *schizophrenic con-fusion* in order to better define the schizophrenic experience of adhesiveness to and intrusiveness from other people, particularly if the individual perceives these people as significant others. In more transactional analytic terms, con-fusion in schizophrenia is considered here to be derived from a structural (i.e., historical) pathology of the Child's experience called *self-fragmentation*, that is, the disorganization and lack of coherence in the experience of the self as a result of early and enduring relational traumas. As such, schizophrenia involves significant transformations in the structure of the intrapsychic (through splitting and body-mind dissociation) as well as relational (through transference-countertransference enactments) experience of the Child-self.

The other comes first

The third assumption is that coming to life as human beings, since the beginning of our intrauterine life, is an act of the Other. Therefore, we are born because of and for the Other. Later on, whatever our body-self (C_0) feels and experiences through the senses in early life can never be meaningfully separated from the responses such a neonatal and infantile ego will elicit from the Other (P_0). This, in turn, will shape the baby's earliest sense of his or her emergent identity (A_0).

Strictly speaking, in the same way that the baby cannot be conceived of as separate from its various relationships with his or her significant others (Winnicott, 1960), there is no such thing as a "schizophrenic ego." There will be, instead, a person whose schizophrenia manifests solely in a relational context. But, because our real parents are there even before we are born, our future life as individuals will depend on their choices and attitudes toward us as infants and in response to our temperament. Thus, as a relational entity, schizophrenia arguably represents a desperate call for personal as well as social responsibility that ultimately means becoming oneself through reference others and allowing the others to become the Others through being ourselves.

The body is the actual theater of the unconscious

From birth and even before, in the prenatal period, our psychic life rests on bodily foundations. As such, our first sense of an ego is a body-ego or, in transactional analysis terms, a Somatic Child (C_1). Nevertheless, following on from the last assumption about the primacy of the Other, this body-ego is by no means restricted to the body and its anatomy. Instead, as a transactional entity available throughout development, this body-ego inevitably carries the traces of the Other. These traces represent a living incarnation of what remains of a variety of actual interactions that took place between the real child and his or her reference people. These earliest memories and representations of the infantile transactions between the subject's emerging ego and the Other(s) are laid down at the multisensory, motor, visceral, organismic (meaning also physiological), preverbal, and nonconscious level. More specifically, by introducing the idea of protocol, Berne conveyed a sense of an inscription on the body of these nonconscious (including creative and intuitive) as well as unconscious (i.e., traumatic) relational (yet symbiotic) experiences that occur very early in life.

Individuals with schizophrenia often elude, refuse, or even reinvent symbolic (i. e., linguistic and imaginative) communication, but cannot escape this subsymbolic, tissue-level of experience of the other. In fact, it becomes inscripted and reinscripted in and through the body without a reflective consciousness. Similarly, in the analytic situation, patient and analyst, through their protocols, both reenact (from the past) and transact (in the present) unconscious and nonconscious dynamics of interbodily reciprocity. Protocol analysis becomes, therefore, the real cure for schizophrenic predicaments.

26

Real cure deserves care and time

The patients described in this book and whom clinical psychiatry currently considers to be "schizophrenic" look very different from those who have been depicted elsewhere as mythical figures venerated by psychiatrists (Szasz, 1961, 1976), sublime subjects (Laing, 1959, 1983 [1967]), somehow romantic figures of modernity (Foucault, 1976; Sass, 1992), representatives of "the sickness of today's society" (Deleuze, 2006, p. 28), and even the most extreme exemplars of the postmodern world (Peters, 2010). Rather, they are individuals whose psychobiography is often marked by premature and enduring traumatic relational experiences with significant others (e.g., parents or other figures acting in *loco parentis*) that lead to the most pervasive fragmentation of the self.

As such, it is of paramount importance that active analytic work is delivered intensively in the contingent setting, be it a hospital, outpatient, or even home setting, with the deliberate purpose of offering patients—and, when possible, also their caregivers—as much time as possible for transforming their schizophrenic breakdown into a breakthrough that will regenerate them from within, meaning also from within their ordinary microsocial and family milieu and hopefully for the rest of their lives.

This is best achieved when transactional analysis, or any other intensive analytic treatment, can be provided, preferably through early multidisciplinary interventions, to psychotic individuals and their caregivers. Acting early and intensively is crucial because first episodes of schizophrenia usually occur during late adolescence or early adulthood, when patients' cognitive, affective, and sociorelational resources are potentially wide-ranging and diversified. In addition, the brain plasticity of these young people may allow effective change in the psychological and neurobiological course of such a disorder in the mind and brain, change that remains developmental but not inevitably neurodegenerative or regressive in essence.

Notes

1 Different theoretical directions in TA developed after Berne, each in relation to a specific theoretical notion of the Adult ego state: Eric Berne's classical model of the personality, later appropriately reinstituted by Stewart and Joines (1987, 2011), was joined over the years by the integrative model of Erskine (1997, 2015), the psychoanalytic model of Moiso and Novellino (2000; Novellino and Moiso, 1990), the constructivist model (Allen & Allen, 1997), the relational model of Hargaden and Sills (2002), the sociocognitive model of Scilligo (2009, 2011), and the cocreative model of Summers and Tudor (2000, 2014a, 2014b), just to mention the main ones. Since we are unable to go into the theoretical-methodological details of each of these models in this book, I argue that Berne's conception of the Adult ego state (Berne 1975b [1961]) is still surprisingly modern and in line with the latest advances in cognitive and affective neuroscience. For me, in fact, the Adult ego state is what connects the whole of Berne's theory of ego states to the biology of the human nervous system, as it is the Adult—understood as A_2 but also as the Adult in the Child (A_1) and Adult in the Parent (A_3)—which is the interface (also neurological)

between the external relational world and the intrapsychic world, thus giving bio-logical substance to the so-called three "psychic organs" (Berne, 1975b [1961]) (the latter classified by Berne into archaeopsyche, exteropsyche, and neopsyche). If we are able to discuss the psychic organs, it is because the only ego state that can be traced back to all three psychic organs as interdependent neurobiological systems (or subsystems) is the Adult in its psychodevelopmental classifications of A_0, A_1, A_2, A_3, An (where "n" stands for umpteenth). In fact, the Adult in various stages of development has both a neurological architecture—that is, one that corresponds to a kind of neuroanatomical logic provided by the development of the central and peripheral nervous systems—and a neuroplasticity that can make psychic organs develop throughout life as experience-dependent biological structures.

2 This functional representation of an ego state in Berne (1975c [1972]) has some-times retained a descriptive character, while in other cases it has ended up almost corresponding to a second model with which to interpret the personality, thereby creating quite a few theoretical disagreements among transactional analysts.

References

Adler, A. (2011). *The practice and the theory of individual psychology.* London: Rou-tledge. (Original work published 1924)

Allen, J. R., & Allen, B. A. (1997). A new type of transactional analysis and one ver-sion of script work with a constructivist sensibility. *Transactional Analysis Journal,* 27, 89–98.

Ashby, W. R. (1950). A new mechanism which shows simple conditioning. *Journal of Psychology,* 29, 343–347.

Bateman, A., Brown, D., & Pedder, J. (2009). *Introduction to psychotherapy: An out-line of principles and practice.* London: Routledge. (Original work published 1979)

Bateson, G. (1956). The message "This is play." In B. Schaffner (Ed.), *Group processes: Transactions of second conference* (pp. 145–242). New York, NY: Josiah Macy, Jr. Foundation.

Berne, E. (1969). *A layman's guide to psychiatry and psychoanalysis.* London: Andre Deutsch. (Original work published 1957)

Berne, E. (1970). *Sex in human loving.* New York, NY: Penguin Books.

Berne, E. (1975a). *The structure and dynamics of organizations and groups.* New York, NY: Grove Press. (Original work published 1963)

Berne, E. (1975b). *Transactional analysis in psychotherapy: A systematic individual and social psychiatry.* London: Souvenir Press. (Original work published 1961)

Berne, E. (1975c). *What do you say after you say hello? The psychology of human destiny.* London: Corgi. (Original work published 1972)

Berne, E. (1977a). Concerning the nature of communication. In E. Berne, P. McCor-mick (Ed.), *Intuition and ego states: The origins of transactional analysis,* pp. 49–64. San Francisco, CA: TA Press. (Original work published 1953)

Berne, E. (1977b). Concerning the nature of diagnosis. In E. Berne, P. McCormick (Ed.), *Intuition and ego states: The origins of transactional analysis,* pp. 33–48. San Francisco, CA: TA Press. (Original work published 1952)

Berne, E. (1977c). Primal images and primal judgment. In E. Berne, P. McCormick (Ed.), *Intuition and ego states: The origins of transactional analysis,* pp. 67–97. San Francisco, CA: TA Press. (Original work published 1955)

Berne, E. (1977d). *Principles of group treatment*. New York, NY: Grove Press. (Original work published 1966)

Berne, E. (1977e). The nature of intuition. In E. Berne, P. McCormick (Ed.), *Intuition and ego states: The origins of transactional analysis*, pp. 1–30. San Francisco, CA: TA Press. (Original work published 1949)

Berne, E. (2008). *Games people play: The psychology of human relationships*. New York, NY: Grove Press. (Original work published 1964)

Bollas, C. (1987). *The shadow of the object: Psychoanalysis of the unthought known*. New York, NY: Columbia University Press.

Bollas, C. (1989). *Forces of destiny: Psychoanalysis and human idiom*. Northvale, NJ: Jason Aronson.

Bowlby, J. (1988). *A secure base: Parent-child attachment and healthy human development*. London: Routledge.

Breuer, J., & Freud, S. (1955). Studies in hysteria. In J. Strachey (Ed. & Trans.), *The standard edition of the complete psychological works of Sigmund Freud* (Vol. 2, pp. 1–335). London: Hogarth Press. (Original work published 1895)

Bucci, W. (1997). *Psychoanalysis and cognitive science: A multiple code theory*. New York, NY: Guilford.

Bucci, W. (2008). The role of bodily experience in emotional organization: New perspectives on the multiple code theory. In F. S. Anderson (Ed.), *Bodies in treatment: The unspoken dimension* (pp. 51–76). New York, NY: The Analytic Press.

Caizzi, C. (2012). Embodied trauma: Using the subsymbolic mode to access and change script protocol in traumatized adults. *Transactional Analysis Journal*, 42, 165–175.

Campbell, J. (2008). *The hero with a thousand faces*. Novato, CA: New World Library. (Original work published 1949)

Cornell, W. F. (2005). In the terrain of the unconscious: The evolution of a transactional analysis therapist. *Transactional Analysis Journal*, 35, 119–131.

Cornell, W. F. (2010). Aspiration or adaptation? An unresolved tension in Eric Berne's basic beliefs. *Transactional Analysis Journal*, 40, 243–253.

Cornell, W. F. (2015a). Play at your own risk: Games, play and intimacy. *Transactional Analysis Journal*, 45, 70–90.

Cornell, W. F. (2015b). *Somatic experience in psychoanalysis and psychotherapy: In the expressive language of the living*. London: Routledge.

Cornell, W. F. (2016). How do we get there from here? Modes of intervention in TA. In W. F. Cornell, A. de Graaf, T. Newson & M. Thunnissen (Eds.), *Into TA: A comprehensive book on transactional analysis* (pp. 201–285). London: Karnac Books.

Cornell, W. F., & Landaiche, N. M., III. (2006). Impasse and intimacy: Applying Berne's concept of script protocol. *Transactional Analysis Journal*, 36, 196–213.

Cornell, W. F., & Landaiche, N. M., III. (2008). Nonconscious processes and self-development: Key concepts from Eric Berne and Christopher Bollas. *Transactional Analysis Journal*, 38, 200–218.

Deleuze, G. (2006). *Two regimes of madness: Texts and interviews 1975–1995*. New York, NY: Semiotext(e).

Deutsch, H. (1942). Some forms of emotional disturbance and their relationship to schizophrenia. *Psychoanalytic Quarterly*, 11, 301–321.

Erikson, E. (1963). *Youth: Change and challenge*. New York, NY: Basic Books.

Erikson, E. (1993). *Childhood and society.* New York, NY: Norton. (Original work published 1950)

Erskine, R. G. (1997). *Theories and methods of an integrative transactional analysis: A volume of select articles.* San Francisco, CA: TA Press.

Erskine, R. G. (2015). *Relational patterns, therapeutic presence: Concepts and practice of integrative psychotherapy.* London: Karnac Books.

Fairbairn, W. R. D. (1952). *An object-relations theory of the personality.* New York, NY: Basic Books.

Federn, P. (1953). *Ego psychology and the psychoses.* London: Imago Publishing. (Original work published 1952)

Foucault, M. (1976). *Mental illness and psychology.* New York, NY: Harper & Row.

Freud, A. (1965). *Normality and pathology in childhood: Assessments of development.* New York, NY: International Universities Press.

Freud, S. (1955a). *A difficulty in the path of psycho-analysis.* In J. Strachey (Ed. & Trans.), *The standard edition of the complete psychological works of Sigmund Freud* (Vol. 17, pp. 135–144). London: Hogarth Press. (Original work published 1917)

Freud, S. (1955b). *Beyond the pleasure principle, group psychology and other works.* In J. Strachey (Ed. & Trans.), *The standard edition of the complete psychological works of Sigmund Freud* (Vol. 18). London: Hogarth Press. (Original work published 1920)

Guglielmotti, R. L. (2008). The quality of the therapeutic relationship as a factor in helping to change the client's protocol or implicit memory. *Transactional Analysis Journal,* 38, 101–109.

Hargaden, H., & Sills, C. (2002). *Transactional analysis: A relational perspective.* Hove: Brunner-Routledge.

Harlow, H. F., & Harlow, M. K. (1962). Social deprivation in monkeys. *Scientific American,* 207, 136–146.

Hartmann, H. (1939). *Ego psychology and the problem of adaptation.* New York, NY: International Universities Press.

Hine, J. (1990). The bilateral and ongoing nature of games. *Transactional Analysis Journal,* 20, 28–39.

Huizinga, J. (2016). *Homo ludens.* Tacoma, WA: Angelico Press. (Original work published 1938)

Janet, P. (1889). *L'automatisme psychologique* [Psychological automatism]. Paris: Félix Alcan.

Janet, P. (1908). L'analyse psychologique et la critique des méthodes de psychothérapie [Psychological analysis and critique of psychotherapeutic methods]. *Annuaire du Collège de France,* 8, 70–71.

Jung, C. G. (2016). *Psychological types.* London: Routledge. (Original work published 1921)

Kierkegaard, S. (1968). *The concept of irony, with continual reference to Socrates* (L. M. Capel, Trans.). Bloomington, IN: Indiana University Press. (Original work published 1841)

Kierkegaard, S. (1991). *Stages on life's way: Studies by various persons* (H. V. Hong & E. H. Hong, Eds. & Trans.). Princeton, NJ: Princeton University Press. (Original work published 1845)

Klein, M. (1952). The origins of transference. *International Journal of Psycho-Analysis,* 33, 433–438.

Klein, M. (1997a). Envy and gratitude. In M. Klein, *Envy and gratitude and other works, 1946–1963* (pp. 176–235). London: Vintage. (Original work published 1957)

Klein, M. (1997b). Some theoretical conclusion regarding the emotional life of the infant. In M. Klein, *Envy and gratitude and other works, 1946–1963* (pp. 61–93). London: Vintage. (Original work published 1952)

Klein, M. (1997c). *The psycho-analysis of children.* London: Vintage. (Original work published 1932)

Laing, R. D. (1959). *The divided self: An existential study in sanity and madness.* London: Penguin Books.

Laing, R. D. (1983). *The politics of experience.* New York, NY: Pantheon Books. (Original work published 1967)

Levine, S. (1960). Stimulation in infancy. *Scientific American,* 202, 80–86.

Ligabue, S. (2007). Being in relationship: Different languages to understand ego states, script, and the body. *Transactional Analysis Journal,* 37, 294–306.

Lorenz, K. Z. (1952). *King Solomon's ring* (M. K. Wilson, Trans.). London: Methuen.

Mahler, M., Pine, F., & Bergman, A. (1975). *The psychological birth of the human infant.* New York, NY: Basic Books.

Moiso, C., & Novellino, M. (2000). An overview of the psychodynamic school of transactional analysis and its epistemological foundations. *Transactional Analysis Journal,* 30, 182–187.

Novak, E. T. (2015). Are games, enactments, and reenactments similar? No, yes, it depends. *Transactional Analysis Journal,* 45, 117–127.

Novellino, M., & Moiso, C. (1990). The psychodynamic approach to transactional analysis. *Transactional Analysis Journal,* 20, 187–192.

Peters, J. D. (2010). Broadcasting and schizophrenia. *Media, Culture & Society,* 32, 123–140.

Pierini, A. (2008). Has the unconscious moved house? *Transactional Analysis Journal,* 38, 110–118.

Rank, O. (2015). *The myth of the birth of the hero: A psychological exploration of the myth.* Baltimore, MD: John Hopkins University Press. (Original work published 1909)

Ruesch, J., & Bateson, G. (1951). *Communication: The social matrix of psychiatry.* New York, NY: Norton.

Sass, L. A. (1992). *Madness and modernism: Insanity in the light of modern art, literature and thought.* Cambridge, MA: Harvard University Press.

Scilligo, P. (2009). *Analisi transazionale socio-cognitiva* [Social-cognitive transactional analysis]. Rome: LAS.

Scilligo, P. (2011). Transference as a measurable social-cognitive process: An application of Scilligo's model of ego states. *Transactional Analysis Journal,* 41, 196–205.

Spitz, R. (1945). Hospitalism: Genesis of psychiatric conditions in early childhood. *Psychoanalytic Study of the Child,* 1, 53–74.

Stern, D. N. (1985). *The interpersonal world of the infant: A view from psychoanalysis and developmental psychology.* New York, NY: Basic Books.

Stern, D. N. (1990). *Diary of a baby.* New York, NY: Basic Books.

Stern, D. N. (1995). *The motherhood constellation: A unified view of parent-infant psychotherapy.* New York, NY: Basic Books.

Stewart, I., & Joines, V. (1987). *TA today: A new introduction to transactional analysis.* Nottingham, and Chapel Hill, NC: Lifespace Publishing.

Stewart, I., & Joines, V. (2011). TA tomorrow. *Transactional Analysis Journal,* 41, 221–229.

Stuthridge, J. (2015). Games, enactment, and countertransference. *Transactional Analysis Journal*, 45, 104–116.

Stuthridge, J., & Sills, C. (2016). Psychological games and intersubjective processes. In R. G. Erskine (Ed.), *Transactional analysis in contemporary psychotherapy* (pp. 185–208). London: Karnac Books.

Summers, G., & Tudor, K. (2000). Cocreative transactional analysis. *Transactional Analysis Journal*, 30, 23–40.

Summers, G., & Tudor, K. (2014a). Co-creative transactional analysis. In K. Tudor & G. Summers (Eds.), *Co-creative transactional analysis: Papers, responses, dialogues, and developments* (pp. 1–28). London: Karnac Books.

Summers, G., & Tudor, K. (2014b). Introducing co-creative transactional analysis. In K. Tudor & G. Summers (Eds.), *Co-creative transactional analysis: Papers, responses, dialogues, and developments* (pp. 235–250). London: Karnac Books.

Szasz, T. (1961). *The myth of mental illness: Foundations of a theory of personal conduct.* New York, NY: Hoeber-Harper.

Szasz, T. (1976). *Schizophrenia: The sacred symbol of psychiatry.* New York, NY: Basic Books.

Walter, W. G. (1950). An imitation of life. *Scientific American*, 182, 42–45.

Walter, W. G. (1951). A machine that learns. *Scientific American*, 185, 60–63.

Watzlawick, P., Beavin, J., & Jackson, D. D. (1967). *Pragmatics of human communication: A study of interactional patterns, pathologies, and paradoxes.* New York, NY: Norton.

Weiss, E. (1950). *Principles of psychodynamics.* New York, NY: Grune & Stratton.

Wiener, N. (1948). Time, communication, and the nervous system. *Annuals of the New York Academy of Science*, 50, 197–220.

Winnicott, D. W. (1960). The theory of the parent-infant relationship. *International Journal of Psychoanalysis*, 41, 585–595.

Winnicott, D. W. (1965). *The maturational processes and the facilitating environment: Studies in a theory of emotional development.* Madison, CT: International Universities Press.

2

SCHIZOPHRENIA OR
SCHIZOPHRENIAS?

A brief history of psychiatric nosography

Schizophrenia is, without question, one of the major psychotic disorders, whose usual onset is in late adolescence and early adulthood. Its phenomenology is characterized by alterations in behavior, thinking, and affectivity along with the presence of what are widely described as "negative" symptoms (e.g., lack of volition, poverty of speech, apathy, minimal or nearly absent social functioning, etc.) and/or "positive" symptoms (e.g., hallucinations, delusions, etc.).

More specifically, the positive symptoms are so called because they represent significant changes in thinking, affectivity, and/or behavior that the person with schizophrenia did not have before he or she became unwell. Negative symptoms indicate, instead, disruptions to thoughts, feelings, and/or behavior that the person used to have before he or she became psychotic but now no longer have or have to a lesser extent and so have been lost or taken away from his or her psyche. As such, this classification rather reductively suggests that something is added to ("positive") or lost from ("negative") the psyche of the person facing a psychotic breakdown. It does not take into account the vibrant complexity of the inner world of the person with schizophrenia, regardless of the type of diagnostic category such complexity may attract by following a mere list of signs and symptoms. By contrast, contemporary transactional analysis can offer a much broader conceptual framework for the in-depth understanding of the predicaments of patients facing schizophrenia with the ultimate aim to develop a more articulate yet integrative and ethically sound psychotherapeutic approach to these persons even in the midst of a psychotic crisis.

Since Berne's original observations of the psychotic process, there has been limited and, at times, problematic attention paid in transactional analysis to the understanding and treatment of schizophrenia. It is the intention of this chapter to provide a brief history of the evolving, and often conflicting, efforts to comprehend and treat this devastating disorder and engage the reader in a deepening awareness of the nature of these life-altering disturbances.

33

The first accounts

The first clinical descriptions of this disorder appear in 1800 and are associated with Philippe Pinel, a psychiatrist at the Salpêtrière Hospital in Paris. His observations are roughly contemporaneous with those of John Haslam, who in 1809 gave a detailed description of a clinical case at the Bethlem Hospital in London, one that would today be deemed a schizophrenic psychosis. Pinel (1806 [1801]) also defined a type of mental alienation as dementia, which was characterized by "rapid succession or uninterrupted alternation of insulated ideas, and evanescent and unconnected emotions. Continually repeated acts of extravagance: complete forgetfulness of every previous state: diminished sensibility to external impressions: abolition of the faculty of judgement: perpetual activity" (p. 164). More accurate still is the description of chronic dementia given to the condition by Etienne Esquirol in his 1838 treatise *Des maladies mentales* (Esquirol, 1845 [1838]). In his opinion, this was caused by excessive masturbation, the abuse of pleasures, and intense intellectual activity. He defined it as "a cerebral affection, ordinarily chronic, and without fever; characterized by disorders of sensibility, understanding, intelligence, and will" (Esquirol, 1845 [1838], p. 21).

The term dementia was later used again by Benedict Augustine Morel (1857), who, in his *Traité des dégénésescence physiques, intellectuelles et morales de l'espèce humaine* (Treaty of the physical, intellectual and moral degenerates of the human species), specified it further with the term démence précoce (dementia praecox) to describe the clinical onset of the condition in an adolescent boy. Wilhelm Sander (1868) reintroduced the word paranoia (as originally given by Hippocrates) to suggest a morbid mental framework based on the delusion of persecution, that is, an altered interpretation of reality whereby individuals believe themselves to be in some way assailed by social events or dynamics in a negative and persecutory way. Ewald Hecker (1871) subsequently use the term hebephrenia (from the Greek Hebe, goddess of youth) to redefine a form of psychosis beginning in adolescence and characterized by alterations in affectivity, childish behaviors, and symptoms of mental weakness. Then in his 1874 monograph, Karl Ludwig Kahlbaum described catatonia as a cyclical condition characterized by stereotyped movements, waxy flexibility, negativism, stupor, and occasional episodes of intense psychomotor agitation.

It was not until 1896 that Emil Kraepelin gave the name dementia praecox to a single condition of severe mental suffering that combined the three forms just mentioned (paranoia, hebephrenia, and catatonia), thereby establishing them within the same disease. In this way, dementia praecox was distinguished in origin from dementia in the elderly because of its onset in youth (hence the adjective "praecox"). Its chronic progression, as assumed at the time, led to a pervasive and persistent decline in the cognitive, affective, and relational life of the person (dementia).

34

Some years after Kraepelin's unifying definition, Swiss psychiatrist Eugen Bleuler boldly proposed renaming this disorder as a group of schizophrenias. In his monograph, entitled *Dementia Praecox oder die Gruppe der Schizofrenien* (Dementia praecox or the group of schizophrenias), Bleuler (1950 [1911]) wrote:

> By the term "dementia praecox" or "schizophrenia" we designate a group of psychoses whose course is at times chronic, at times marked by intermittent attacks, and which can stop or retrograde at any stage. ... The disease is characterized by a specific type of alteration of thinking, feeling and relation to the external world which appear nowhere else in this particular fashion. ... Thus the process of association often works with mere fragments of ideas and concepts. ... In the severest cases emotional and affective expressions seem completely lacking. In milder cases we may note only the degree of intensity of the emotional reactions is not commensurate with the various events that caused those reactions. Indeed, the intensity of the affective reactions may range from a complete lack of emotional expression to extremely exaggerated affective responses in relation to different thought-complexes. They affectively can also appear to be qualitatively abnormal; that is, inadequate to the intellectual processes involved. In addition to the often-discussed signs of "deterioration," many other symptoms are present in a majority of the hospital cases. We find hallucinations, delusions, confusion, stupor, mania and melancholic affective fluctuations, and catatonic symptoms.
>
> (pp. 8–12)

Bleuler's definition indicates the heterogeneity of the clinical phenomenology of this disorder. He justified his choice of the term schizophrenia rather than dementia praecox arguing that Zerreissung (i.e., the tearing apart leading to fragmentation of self experience) or Spaltung (splitting) of psychic functions were "the prominent symptoms" of this disorder (Bleuler, 1987 [1908], p. 59). Among the many symptoms he described, Bleuler believed that the loosening of associations, alterations in affectivity, autism, and ambivalence (later reduced to the mnemonic known as Bleuler's four "A"s) to be fundamental.

Kurt Schneider (1959), another European psychiatrist, also contributed to a subsequent conceptualization of schizophrenia similarly based on symptoms. Like Bleuler, Schneider focused on the identification of "first-rank symptoms" (including auditory hallucinations in the form of voices in dialogue or voices as commentary, thought echo, thought insertion/withdrawal/broadcasting, delusions of somatic influence and control, etc.) deemed by him to be characteristic of the schizophrenic disorder. In fact, these symptoms are no longer considered pathognomonic of the schizophrenic condition because they are found in the broader spectrum of psychotic and dissociative disorders.

35

Each of these authors naturally emphasized symptoms or aspects of schizophrenic psychosis based on their own clinical observations and beliefs about the origin of the disorder, although their descriptions were not supported by clear biological evidence.

Nevertheless, Kraepelin's, Bleuler's, and Schneider's perspectives on schizophrenia still coexist in contemporary psychiatric classifications of this major mental disorder as set out in the *Diagnostic and statistical manual of mental disorders* (American Psychiatric Association, 2000, 2013) and the *International classification of diseases* (World Health Organization, 1992). From the 1960s onward, and in the wake of dissent raised by antipsychiatry forces (Laing, 1959; Szasz, 1961, 1976) about the predominantly biological view of schizophrenia, a disconcerting, to put it mildly, number of hypotheses and interpretations about the origin of this condition have appeared. These have contributed to further confusion about the meaning, boundaries, and even the clinical value of the original term schizophrenia. This nosographic confusion has not yet been resolved because there is still no common view of the etiological and pathogenetic mechanisms of this psychiatric condition. It therefore cannot be considered an illness but is viewed as a syndrome, that is, as a group of nonspecific signs and symptoms strongly associated with each other.

Contemporary psychiatry also continues to fluctuate between a categorical view of schizophrenic psychosis based on symptoms (delusions, hallucinations, alterations in affectivity, disorders of thought and behavior, etc.) and a dimensional view based on dimensions or clusters of symptoms linked to a shared alteration of function and an assumed specific physiopathological mechanism (e.g., transformation of reality, ideoaffective impoverishment, disorganization, etc.).

The neurobiological evidence and its discontents

The neurodegenerative model of schizophrenia

To date, the fundamental pathobiology of the schizophrenic disorder remains elusive, despite the proliferation of complex explanatory models produced by neuroscience in which much of the evidence from brain pathology, structural and functional neuroimaging, genetics, neuropsychology, and gene-environment interaction studies is set within more or less coherent and thought-provoking theoretical frameworks. In science, there is still a question about the existence of a neurodegenerative—or, conversely, a neurodevelopmental— process that can explain certain neurobiological aspects of schizophrenia.

A contributing role of neurodegeneration in the physiopathology of schizophrenia—in line with Kraepelin's original observations—is, in fact, a focus of contemporary neuroscience research. Neurodegeneration may explain the long latency period before the onset of symptoms, the heterogeneous but mostly disabling clinical course of the disease, the fact that many patients are faced with different degrees of cognitive and behavioral decline, and the partial effectiveness of pharmacological treatment in modifying the course of the disorder.

Neurodegenerative diseases are defined as chronic and progressive disorders of the nervous system that alter neurological and behavioral functions because of specific biochemical changes that are responsible for histopathological alterations and distinct clinical syndromes (Hardy & Gwinn-Hardy, 1998). These diseases include Alzheimer's, Huntington's, Parkinson's, Wilson's, and spongiform encephalopathies (such as Creutzfeld-Jakob disease). Most of these have genetic bases with various transmission modes, but, compared with them, schizophrenia does not have a clear genetic transmissibility nor does it present pathognomonic histopathological features. Nevertheless, neuroimaging studies based on increasingly sophisticated methodologies and techniques have made it possible to trace the course of specific brain changes associated with schizophrenia, highlighting the progressive loss of cortical tissue as well as the enlargement of the cerebral ventricles (DeLisi et al., 1997; Ho et al., 2003; Mathalon et al., 2001).

The neurodevelopmental model of schizophrenia

Whereas Kraepelin's idea of dementia praecox suggested a premature and progressive brain degeneration, others have viewed schizophrenia as a neurodevelopmental disorder in which structural brain changes caused by an early perinatal or even prenatal insult create a predisposition toward the development of the disorder without, however, causing neurodegeneration. Instead, brain development follows the normal processes of maturation and brain aging (Murray, 1994; Murray & Lewis, 1987; Weinberger, 1986; Weinberger & Marenco, 2003). According to the neurodevelopmental hypothesis, the etiology of schizophrenia may involve pathological processes caused by both genetic and environmental factors whose influences begin before the brain reaches its anatomical maturation during adolescence and early adulthood (Dean et al., 2003; Rapoport et al., 2005).

This theory postulates the alteration of normal neuronal development in specific areas and neuronal circuits that results in a brain malfunction. These alterations are not degenerative, per se, and do not cause immediate clinical signs such as those that occur in other disorders such as autism, fragile X syndrome, or Down syndrome. Instead, these alterations present after a latency period that varies between 1 and 3 decades. The events that trigger the onset of the disorder are not fully understood but are believed to include normal neurobiological maturation processes (e.g., neuronal and glial proliferation and migration, axonal and dendritic cell proliferation, apoptosis, axonal myelination, synaptic pruning) that interact with environmental factors (e.g., exposure to gestational insults such as traumas of various kinds, infections, substance abuse, etc.).

The integrative approach in neurobiological models

Subsequent studies on the neurobiological aspects of schizophrenia, in different areas of neuroscientific research, have led certain authors to reconsider the dichotomy between neurodevelopment and neurodegeneration as part of the same pathogenic, two-phase trajectory (Church et al., 2002; McClure & Lieberman, 2003). As a result, this integrative model argues for an interactive process between a neurodevelopmental vulnerability and a progressive deterioration associated with neurotoxicity (Mathalon et al., 2003). According to this view, it appears that certain brain anomalies precede the onset of schizophrenic psychosis, whereas others are associated with the onset itself. There is biological evidence of the deterioration of these anomalies during the course of the disorder. However, it is still not clear whether these anomalies constitute ongoing developmental changes that characterize late adolescence and early adulthood; whether they, in fact, indicate a degenerative change; or whether they are actually due to antipsychotic treatment (Dazzan et al., 2005; Murray & Dean, 2008). To all this we can add the interweaving of a series of neurotransmitter hypotheses relating to the famous hypothesis of dopaminergic dysregulation (Carlsson & Lindqvist, 1963; Kapur, 2003; Laruelle et al., 1996) and subsequent glutamatergic and GABA-ergic hypotheses, without now sparing any of the well-known neurotransmitters in the neurochemical arena.

Whether there are specific brain regions and neural circuits involved in the pathogenesis of schizophrenia, or whether, instead, there is a widespread neurobiological alteration, remains unclear. Some authors have actually hypothesized that schizophrenia is a disorder of neural disconnectivity (Andreasen, 1999) and that, as a result, changes in the brain, seen in structural and functional neuroimaging, reflect a widespread loss of neural connections as implied by Bleuler (1987 [1908]) with his concept of the "fragmentation of the mind."

There is not room here to explore in depth the key hypotheses and neurobiological models of schizophrenia, enriched over the years by genetic studies, electrophysiology, and most importantly, epigenetics and psycho-neuro-immuno-endocrinology. Instead, I have provided references in this chapter to those authors who have been pioneers in contributing to the development of large-scale research in neuroscience on what is still held to be the "sublime object of psychiatry" (Woods, 2011, p. 8).

The exploration of schizophrenic psychosis as presented here can now be expanded to include psychological, relational, and social-environmental dynamics. I explore them through the epistemological lens of transactional analysis, which is able to interact with the biology of the schizophrenic condition.

The role of relational trauma in schizophrenic psychoses: Between transactional analysis and neuroscience

In the last two decades, interest in the scientific community has increasingly focused on social and psychological factors that show a clear, significant association with the biology of schizophrenia (Bebbington et al., 2004; Miller et al., 2001; Morgan & Fisher, 2007; Read et al., 2005). Among the social and psychological factors deemed able to interact with a genetic vulnerability to schizophrenia are stressful life events, adverse social circumstances, belonging to specific ethnic groups (particularly in migration), the degree of urbanization (often associated with socioeconomic poverty and social isolation), prolonged use of psychotropic substances (cannabis, amphetamines, hallucinogens, etc.), and, interestingly, a history of infantile traumas.

In a review of environmental factors associated with schizophrenia, Morgan and Fisher (2007) wrote:

> One consequence of the recent rapid advances in the neurosciences and genetics is that we are beginning to understand how social experience across the life course interacts with genes, and impacts on biological development, to shape adult outcomes. These insights are now being used to produce biological models linking adverse social experiences, including childhood trauma, and adult psychosis.
>
> (p. 8)

In a more recent article published in *Schizophrenia Bulletin*, the internationally renowned psychiatrist Sir Robin Murray (2017)—professor of psychiatric research at the Institute of Psychiatry, Psychology and Neuroscience at King's College in London and one of the most influential scientists in schizophrenia research—admitted that for too long he ignored social factors that contribute to schizophrenia. He also reported that he neglected the negative effects of antipsychotic medications on the brain. Murray wrote:

> Amazingly, such is the power of the Kraepelinian model that some psychiatrists still refuse to accept the evidence, and cling to the nihilistic view that there exists an intrinsically progressive schizophrenic process, a view greatly to the detriment of their patients.
>
> (p. 254)

In contrast, transactional analysis has based its theory of personality and psychopathology on the what, how, when, and how long that characterize individuals' life experiences in their multiple relationships with real and significant reference figures and more generally with the surrounding environment. Unparalleled in its originality—as well as being in line with the Eriksonian psychoanalytic tradition, on the one hand, and contemporary neuroscience, on the other—is Eric Berne's idea of cumulative trauma, which is able to generate psychopathology. To illustrate this idea, in *Transactional analysis in psychotherapy*, Berne (1975a [1961]) created a striking and effective metaphor to explain the development of the personality in conditions of health as well as psychopathology: the metaphor of the coins. He compared a person's psychic balance to a pile of coins in which each coin is the product of a whole range of everyday experiences (e.g., thoughts, emotions, behaviors, somatic experiences, etc.) that correspond with ego states. Consistent with this metaphor, it follows that to accumulate traumatic experiences means to accumulate warped coins and therefore dysfunctional ego states. The nature of the trauma, as well as the number of significant traumas, experienced by individuals during their development can seriously endanger mental health, like a pile of coins that is out of alignment, skewed, wavering, or even about to topple over. Berne clearly bestowed a psychodevelopmental view on this metaphor explaining the pathogenesis of mental disorders when he wrote this:

> The lower down the warped coin is, the greater its effect on the ultimate stability. At this point, it would be possible to speak of different kinds of coins: the pennies of childhood, the nickels of the latent period, the quarters of adolescence, and the silver dollars of maturity. Here one bent penny might eventually cause thousands of silver dollars to tumble in chaos.
>
> (p. 54)

Therefore, for Berne, traumatic experiences in infancy, if not rectified by subsequent positive experiences, can significantly impact the pathophysiology of mental disorders in the adult.

The metaphor of the coins is particularly useful for helping us to understand the pathogenesis of schizophrenic psychoses by highlighting two crucial aspects: on the one hand, its multifactorial and polytraumatic origin, and on the other, its delayed phenomenological expression compared with the period of the first actual traumatic experiences. Just as a pile of coins preserves at the base of its structure the rift of the first warped pennies, so the personality structure of the psychotic subject carries with it the early and already traumatic experiences of childhood and early adolescence. And just as that pile of coins—about to grow bigger with the most recently added and more valuable coins—collapses when it reaches a certain height, so the personality of the schizophrenic cracks catastrophically during the first psychotic episode, which comes, not surprisingly, just on the threshold of youth and early adulthood.

More specifically, the key notion that informs Berne's (1975a [1961]) transactional analysis of schizophrenic psychoses is that the ego of a schizophrenic person is a weakened one. That is, an ego that in the midst of a psychotic breakdown has lost its structural stability, its internal coherence, its sense of agency in the real world, and, ultimately, its sense of being a personal ego and therefore a self.

The view that the psychotic ego is a weakened one is neither new nor unique to Berne's theory. In fact, it flows from the clinical work and theoretical insights of Berne's own analyst, Paul Federn (1953 [1952]). What is special to Berne is the groundbreaking idea that even the psychotic ego is not an irremediably broken one—or a deeply regressed, primarily narcissistic and inaccessible self—but an ego that is still developing, even though its traumatic and trembling relational foundations might cause it to repeatedly fall to pieces and fragment.

Within this focus, Berne's (1975a [1961]) conceptualization of the Adult ego state as, among the other ego states (Parent and Child), the one actualizing adaptation to the current reality at different stages of neurological and psychological development is still incredibly modern. It provides an invaluable insight into transactional analysis theory and the therapeutic approach to schizophrenic psychoses.

Indeed, Berne's understanding of the Adult as a neopsyche (literally meaning a "new mind") that represents a set of both psychological and neurological structures able to change and reorganize (i.e., renew) themselves throughout life $(A_0, A_1, A_2, A_3, A_n)$, anticipated to a remarkable degree the broader concept of neuroplasticity when applied to the physiology of the human brain. Moreover, Berne's view of the whole ego as an evolving pluripartite organization gives credit and hope to the real possibility that psychotherapy itself—and first and foremost transactional analysis—can even change the course of schizophrenia, a disorder in the mind and brain that remains developmental but not inevitably neurodegenerative or regressive in its essence.

Following Berne's (1975a [1961]) initial description of psychoses, the most well-known contributions in the transactional analysis literature on the subject of psychosis come from work by Schiff (1975) and her colleagues. Schiff's model, however, has been called into question because her theoretical assumptions concerning the nature and treatment of schizophrenic experiences rest on unsubstantiated speculations about the pathogenesis of schizophrenia itself (Cornell et al., 2016, pp. 179–180; Mellacqua, 2014). Such speculations also included much more controversial ideas about the causal influence of invariably negative parenting on individuals suffering from psychosis. As a result, Schiff's methodology has actually proven to be detrimental to patients and their families.

Since the collapse of the Schiffian approach to psychosis, there have been only a few attempts within the transactional analysis literature to further review the theory and treatment of psychotic disorders (Caravella & Marone 2003; English, 1977; Moiso, 1985; Moiso & Novellino, 2000; Novellino, 1990, 1991, 2004a [1998], 2004b). Disconcertingly, it took almost four decades before a more comprehensive approach to the transactional analysis understanding and psychotherapy of psychosis—more precisely schizophrenia (Mellacqua, 2014)—could be developed and cast in a more contemporary light. Indeed, apart from Berne's (1969 [1957]) original observations about the role of different types of splitting as mediating factors in the development of psychosis (described in the clinical case of Cary in Chapter 6 of *A layman's guide to psychiatry and psychoanalysis*), the essential link between the individual's traumatic relational experiences, the processes of exclusion, and schizophrenic psychosis has not been considered and evaluated in depth in the transactional analysis literature. Fortunately, in more recent years, there have been a few significant exceptions coming from the independent work of internationally renowned clinicians such as Cornell (2016) and Stuthridge (2012). In my view, their contributions constitute richly informative attempts to reconceptualize psychotic processes within a transactional analysis perspective. Although not addressing schizophrenia directly, these two authors have provided deeply honest, unprecedented, and challenging inquiries into the nature and treatment of psychotic levels of self-disturbance within the TA frame of reference.

More precisely, Stuthridge's 2012 article, drawing on contemporary relational psychoanalytic theories, offered a clear contribution to the development of a more coherent transactional analysis understanding of the fundamental links existing between trauma, dissociation, and enactment of fragmented parts of the self within and outside the analytic setting. She described clearly how each of us (also as therapists) unconsciously externalize fragments of our internal world through games and enactments and how such dynamics can be potentially informative and even reparative.

On the other hand, Cornell's article illustrates in depth a failed psychotherapy with a patient on the verge of a psychotic breakdown. Through his intensely moving and enriching accounts of his countertransference reactions in the work with Samantha he honestly captured the essence of such a painful and yet very much needed job: that of becoming the analysts of individuals who manifest deep states of psychological and interpersonal disturbance such as those experienced by persons suffering from schizophrenia. This is a work, as Cornell lucidly put it, through which we would ultimately need to find a way to be able to see and confront aspects of our own psychotic thinking and functioning.

Both Cornell's and Stuthridge's articles emphasized what I have personally found in my work with psychotic patients. Therapists' are ultimately responsible for sustaining within themselves—specifically at an unlanguaged protocol level of experience—hatred and love, violence and apathy, conflict and solitude, actual precariousness and uncertainty for the future, and the whole ambiguity of being human that a deeply troubled mind, such as the one of a person with psychosis, is able to potently induce through the therapeutic relationship. Doubtlessly, such an attitude on the part of therapists toward their own protocol analysis and self-examination requires considerable time and personal commitment, as well as often supervision and ongoing personal therapy. This kind of therapeutic process can prove to be more informative and transformative for both the patient and the therapist than methods that use more conscious attunement, inquiry, and empathy.

Returning to Berne

I offer here in Berne's words my final call for the deepening of our exploratory view of schizophrenic psychoses:

> Standing on the small island of the intellect, many are trying to understand the sea of life; at most we can understand only the flotsam and jetsam, the flora and the fauna which are cast upon the shores. Taking a verbal or mechanical microscope to what we find will help but little to know what lies beyond the horizon or in the depths. For this we must swim or dive, even if the prospect dismays us at first.
>
> (Berne, 1977e [1949], p. 28)

Ultimately, Berne's eloquent comment echoes my previous work (Mellacqua, 2014) on this neglected—I might better say "excluded"—area of clinical transactional analysis. I am strongly advocating a return to Berne's early writings on unconscious processes (Berne, 1977e [1949], 1977b [1952], 1977a [1953], 1977c [1955]) and, later, on protocol (Berne, 1975a [1961], 1977d [1966], 1975b [1972]), his incredibly modern view of the impact of cumulative trauma (particularly relational trauma) in altering and shaping psychodevelopment (Berne, 1975a [1961]), and his own sharp reflections on schizophrenia itself, which strikingly emphasized ego state splitting and exclusion (Berne, 1969 [1957], 1975a [1961]). These are, at least in my view, the essence or pillars on which transactional analysts can now build a much more solid as well as articulate body of knowledge and techniques for the understanding and cure of schizophrenic suffering.

References

American Psychiatric Association (2000). *Diagnostic and statistical manual of mental disorders* (4th edn). Washington, DC: APA.

American Psychiatric Association (2013). *Diagnostic and statistical manual of mental disorders* (5th edn). Washington, DC: APA.

Andreasen, N. C. (1999). A unitary model of schizophrenia: Bleuler's "fragmented phrenschizencephaly." *Archives of General Psychiatry*, 56, 781–787.

Bebbington, P. E., Bhugra, D., Bhugra, T., Singleton, N., Farrell, M., Jenkins, R., & Meltzer, H. (2004). Psychosis, victimisation and childhood disadvantage: Evidence from the second British national survey of psychiatric morbidity. *British Journal of Psychiatry*, 185, 220–226.

Berne, E. (1969). *A layman's guide to psychiatry and psychoanalysis.* London: Andre Deutsch. (Original work published 1957)

Berne, E. (1975a). *Transactional analysis in psychotherapy: A systematic individual and social psychiatry.* London: Souvenir Press. (Original work published 1961)

Berne, E. (1975b). *What do you say after you say hello? The psychology of human destiny.* London: Corgi. (Original work published 1972)

Berne, E. (1977a). Concerning the nature of communication. In E. Berne, P. McCormick (Ed. & Trans.), *Intuition and ego states: The origins of transactional analysis* (pp. 49–64). San Francisco, CA: TA Press. (Original work published 1953)

Berne, E. (1977b). Concerning the nature of diagnosis. In E. Berne, P. McCormick (Ed. & Trans.), *Intuition and ego states: The origins of transactional analysis* (pp. 33–48). San Francisco, CA: TA Press. (Original work published 1952)

Berne, E. (1977c). Primal images and primal judgment. In E. Berne, P. McCormick, (Ed. & Trans.), *Intuition and ego states: The origins of transactional analysis* (pp. 67–97). San Francisco, CA: TA Press. (Original work published 1955)

Berne, E. (1977d). *Principles of group treatment*. New York, NY: Grove Press. (Original work published 1966)

Berne, E. (1977e). The nature of intuition. In E. Berne, P. McCormick (Ed. & Trans.), *Intuition and ego states: The origins of transactional analysis* (pp. 1–30). San Francisco, CA: TA Press. (Original work published 1949)

Bleuler, E. (1950). *Dementia praecox or the group of schizophrenias* (Monograph Series on Schizophrenia 1) (J. Zinkin, Trans.). New York, NY: International Universities Press. (Original work published 1911)

Bleuler, E. (1987). The prognosis of dementia praecox: The group of schizophrenias. In J. Cutting & M. Shepherd (Eds.), *The clinical roots of the schizophrenia concept: Translations of seminal European contributions on schizophrenia* (pp. 59–74). Cambridge: Cambridge University Press. (Original work published 1908)

Caravella, M., & Marone, A. (2003). Acute psychotic states: A clinical interpretation. *Transactional Analysis Journal, 33,* 246–253.

Carlsson, A., & Lindqvist, M. (1963). Effect of chlorpromazine or haloperidol on formation of 3methoxytyramine and normetanephrine in mouse brain. *Acta Pharmacology Toxicology, 20,* 140–144.

Church, S. M., Cotter, D., Bramon, E., & Murray, R. M. (2002). Does schizophrenia result from developmental or degenerative processes? *Journal of Neural Transmission Supplementum, 63,* 129–147.

Cornell, W. F. (2016). Failing to Do the Job. *Transactional Analysis Journal, 46,* 266–276.

Cornell, W. F., de Graaf, A., Newton, T., & Thunnissen, M. (2016). *Into TA: A comprehensive textbook of transactional analysis.* London: Karnac Books.

Dazzan, P., Morgan, K. D., Orr, K., Hutchinson, G., Chitnis, X., Suckling, J., Murray, R. M. (2005). Different effects of typical and atypical antipsychotics on grey matter in first episode psychosis: The AESOP study. *Neuropsychopharmacology, 30,* 765–774.

Dean, K., Bramon, E., & Murray, R. M. (2003). The causes of schizophrenia: Neurodevelopment and other risk factors. *Journal of Psychiatric Practice, 9,* 442–454.

DeLisi, L. E., Sakuma, M., Tew, W., Kushner, M., Hoff, A. L., & Grimson, R. (1997). Schizophrenia as a chronic active brain process: A study of progressive brain structural change subsequent to the onset of schizophrenia. *Psychiatry Research, 74,* 129–140.

English, F. (1977). What shall I do tomorrow? Reconceptualizing transactional analysis. In G. Barnes (Ed.), *Transactional analysis after Eric Berne: Teachings and practices of three TA schools* (pp. 287–347). New York, NY: Harper's College Press.

Esquirol, J. E. D. (1845). *Mental maladies: A treatise on insanity* (E. Kingsbury Hunt, Trans.). Philadelphia, PA: Lea and Blanchard. (Original work published 1838)

Federn, P. (1953). *Ego psychology and the psychoses.* London: Imago Publishing. (Original work published 1952)

Hardy, J., & Gwinn-Hardy, K. (1998). Genetic classification of primary neurodegenerative disease. *Science,* 282, 1075–1079.

Hecker, E. (1871). *Hebephrenie* [Hebephrenia]. *Archiv für Pathologische Anatomie und Phisiologie und für Klinische Medizin,* 25, 394–429.

Ho, B. C., Andreasen, N. C., Nopoulos, P., Arndt, S., Magnotta, V., & Flaum, M. (2003). Progressive structural brain abnormalities and their relationships to clinical outcome: A longitudinal magnetic resonance imaging study early in schizophrenia. *Archives of General Psychiatry,* 60, 585–594.

Kahlbaum, K. L. (1874). *Die katatonie oder das spannungsirresein: Eine klinische form psychischer krankheit* [Catatonia or tension insanity: A clinical form of mental illness]. Berlin: Hirschwald.

Kapur, S. (2003). Psychosis as a state of aberrant salience: A framework linking biology, phenomenology, and pharmacology in schizophrenia. *American Journal of Psychiatry,* 160, 13–23.

Kraepelin, E. (1896). *Psychiatrie: Ein Lehrbuch für Studirende und Aerzte* [Psychiatry: A textbook for students and doctors] (5th edn). Leipzig: Barth.

Laing, R. D. (1959). *The divided self: An existential study in sanity and madness.* London: Penguin Books.

Laruelle, M., Abi-Dargham, A., Van Dyck, C. H., Gil, R., D'Souza, C. D., Erdos, J., & Innis, R. B. (1996). Single photon emission computerized tomography imaging of amphetamine-induced dopamine release in drug-free schizophrenic subjects. *Proceedings of the National Academy of Sciences,* 93, 9235–9240.

Mathalon, D. H., Rapoport, J. L., Davis, K. L., & Krystal, J. H. (2003). Neurotoxicity, neuroplasticity, and magnetic resonance imaging morphometry. *Archives of General Psychiatry,* 60, 846–848.

Mathalon, D. H., Sullivan, E. V., Lim, K. O., & Pfefferbaum, A. (2001). *Progressive brain volume changes and the clinical course of schizophrenia in men: A longitudinal magnetic resonance imaging study. Archives of General Psychiatry,* 58, 148–157.

McClure, R. K., & Lieberman, J. A. (2003). Neurodevelopmental and neurodegenerative hypothesis of schizophrenia: A review and critique. *Current Opinion in Psychiatry,* 16, 15–18.

Mellacqua, Z. (2014). Beyond symbiosis: The role of primal exclusions in schizophrenic psychosis. *Transactional Analysis Journal,* 44, 8–30.

Miller, P., Lawrie, S. M., Hodges, A., Clafferty, R., Cosway, R., & Johnstone, E. C. (2001). Genetic liability, illicit drug use, life stress and psychotic symptoms: Preliminary findings from the Edinburgh study of people at high risk for schizophrenia. *Social Psychiatry and Psychiatric Epidemiology,* 36, 338–342.

Moiso, C. (1985). Ego states and transference. *Transactional Analysis Journal,* 15, 194–201.

Moiso, C., & Novellino, M. (2000). An overview of the psychodynamic school of transactional analysis and its epistemological foundations. *Transactional Analysis Journal,* 30, 182–187.

Morel, B. A. (1857). *Traité des dégénérescences physiques, intellectuelles et morales de l'espèce humaine et des causes qui produisent ces variétés maladives* [A treatise on the physical, intellectual and moral degeneration of the human species and the causes that produce these unhealthy varieties]. Paris: J. B. Baillière. [Reprint: New York, NY: Arno Press, 1976]

Morgan, C., & Fisher, H. (2007). Environmental factors in schizophrenia: Childhood trauma, a critical review. *Schizophrenia Bulletin*, 33, 3–10.

Murray, R. M. (1994). Neurodevelopmental schizophrenia: The rediscovery of dementia praecox. *British Journal of Psychiatry*, 25, 6–12.

Murray, R. M. (2017). Mistakes I have made in my research career. *Schizophrenia Bulletin*, 43, 253–256.

Murray, R. M., & Dean, K. (2008). Schizophrenia and related disorders. In R. M. Murray, K. S. Kendler, P. McGuffin, S. Wessely, & D. J. Castle (Eds.), *Essential psychiatry* (pp. 284–319). Cambridge: Cambridge University Press.

Murray, R. M., & Lewis, S. W. (1987). Is schizophrenia a neurodevelopmental disorder? *British Medical Journal*, 296, 681–682.

Novellino, M. (1990). Unconscious communication and interpretation in transactional analysis. *Transactional Analysis Journal*, 20, 168–172.

Novellino, M. (1991). *Psicologia clinica dell'io* [Clinical psychology of the ego]. Rome: Astrolabio.

Novellino, M. (2004a). *Approccio clinico dell'analisi transazionale: Epistemologia, metodologia e psicopatologia clinica* [The clinical approach of transactional analysis: Epistemology, methodology and clinical psychopathology]. Milan: Franco Angeli. (Original work published 1998)

Novellino, M. (2004b). *Psicoanalisi transazionale* [Transactional psychoanalysis]. Milan: Franco Angeli.

Pinel, P. (1806). *A treatise on insanity* (D. Davis, Trans.). London: Cadell & Davis, Strand. (Original work published 1801)

Rapoport, J. L., Addington, A. M., Frangou, S., & Psych, M. R. (2005). The neurodevelopmental model of schizophrenia: Update 2005. *Molecular Psychiatry*, 10, 434–449.

Read, J., Van Os, J., Morrison, A. P., & Ross, C. A. (2005). Childhood trauma, psychosis and schizophrenia: A literature review with theoretical and clinical implications. *Acta Psychiatrica Scandinavica*, 112, 330–350.

Sander, W. (1868). Übereine spezielle form der primären verrücktheit [A special form of primary madness]. *Archiv für Psychiatrie und Nervenkrankheiten*, 1, 387–419.

Schiff, J. L. (with Schiff, A. W., Mellor, K., Schiff, E., Schiff, S., Richman, D., Fishman, J., & Momb, D.) (1975). *Cathexis reader: Transactional analysis treatment of psychosis*. New York, NY: Harper & Row.

Schneider, K. (1959). *Clinical psychopathology* (5th edn). New York, NY: Grune & Stratton.

Stuthridge, J. (2012). Traversing the fault lines: Trauma and enactment. *Transactional Analysis Journal*, 42, 238–251.

Szasz, T. (1961). *The myth of mental illness: Foundations of a theory of personal conduct*. New York, NY: Hoeber-Harper.

Szasz, T. (1976). *Schizophrenia: The sacred symbol of psychiatry*. New York, NY: Basic Books.

Weinberger, D. R. (1986). The pathogenesis of schizophrenia: A neurodevelopmental theory. In H. A. Nasrallah & D. R. Weinberger (Eds.), *The neurology of schizophrenia* (pp. 387–405). Amsterdam: Elsevier.

Weinberger, D. R., & Marenco, S. (2003). Schizophrenia as a neurodevelopmental disorder. In D. R. Weinberger & S. R. Hirsch (Eds.), *Schizophrenia* (pp. 326–348). Oxford: Blackwell Science.

Woods, A. (2011). *The sublime object of psychiatry: Schizophrenia in clinical and cultural theory.* New York, NY: Oxford University Press.

World Health Organization (1992). *The ICD-10 classification of mental and behavioral disorders.* Geneva: WHO.

3

TRANSACTIONAL PSYCHOPATHOLOGY OF SCHIZOPHRENIC PSYCHOSES

Intrapsychic conflict model of schizophrenia: Contaminations, impasses, and symbiosis

Bernean metapsychology includes theoretical elements attributable to both intrapsychic conflict and deficit models of the human psyche and human psychopathology. On the one hand, the structural conflict model can be found in Berne's (1975a [1961], p. 48) formulation of *contamination* between two or among different ego states. On the other, important theoretical nuclei of a deficit model in transactional analysis are evident in what Berne defined, in his structural diagrams, as *exclusion* (p. 46). In fact, conflict and deficit theories coexist in the classical structural model of psychopathology proposed by Berne.

As previously explained (see Chapter 1), in Berne's model of transactional analysis the theoretical propositions attributed to the conflict view as well as those focused on the deficit view of psychopathology find a common position within a broader humanistic-existential philosophical framework (literally a framework of humanism and existentialism). Much of Berne's theoretical corpus is directly inspired by Greek and Latin culture, as shown by his repeated references to classical mythology, and by the existentialism of writers such as Sartre and Kierkegaard, from whom Berne derived his vision of a tragic Man who is not the only maker of his own destiny.

From the beginning of his existence, Berne's Man finds himself actively involved in a continuous narrative of human relationships, consumed deep in his biology by hungers for the Other, his identity shaped by the presence (as well as by the "present" absence) of many Others, he himself being this teeming plurality that results in him being unable to integrate and define himself without recognition of the Other, by the Other, and in the Other. According to this perspective, the individual's intrapsychic and relational life, with its attendant joys and sufferings, seems therefore to unfold out of an existential thread of transactions with significant others and external reality.

There becoming oneself—understood here as autonomy and self-realization—cannot be considered without an interchange of intimacy, that special condition of being open to the other and surrounding reality, simultaneously capturing the wonder and mystery of both.

To return to the subject of schizophrenic psychoses, although an extensive theory and methodology of the role of contamination in psychosis was developed by Berne, there have been only a few theoretical and methodological advances since then about the influence of exclusion within Berne's and post-Bernean transactional analysis, particularly for the understanding of schizophrenia-like psychoses. In contrast, since Berne, the conflict model of psychopathology in transactional analysis has produced invaluable contributions to TA theory and methodology as represented by Goulding and Goulding's (1976, 1979) theory of impasses.

The term *impasse* in the transactional analysis literature is associated with the work of Robert Goulding and Mary Goulding (1976, 1979). They and their early followers (Mellor, 1980) characterized the impasse as an intrapsychic phenomenon, namely, as a conflict between ego states at different stages of psychodevelopment (P_2/C_2, P_1/C_1, P_0/C_0) from which the corresponding terms *type one, type two,* and *type three impasses* originated. They used techniques derived from gestalt therapy, as developed by its founder Fritz Perls (1969), which were embedded within a TA structural theory of psychopathology based essentially on Berne's idea of double contaminations (see Chapter 1).

The Gouldings' theory of impasses provided transactional analysis with a new model for psychotherapeutic intervention called *redecision therapy*. This approach, in its original formulation, is, however, informed by the assumption that the resolution of a patient's intrapsychic conflicts is based on a conscious decision made by the Adult part of the person's personality, with the therapist then being a sort of active facilitator of the whole therapeutic process and, ultimately, of the patient's "change." Much emphasis is thus placed on the potency of the therapist and the therapist's expertise in actively helping the patient take personal responsibility. It often involves a deliberate confrontational approach and avoids working with transference and countertransference in the therapeutic relationship.

More specifically, as regards the structural analysis of schizophrenia, Goulding and Goulding (1979, Chapter 2) suggested a model of complex contaminations—the triple contamination—to explain the phenomenology of psychosis. In my view, this model not only looks too simplistic but is also not even based on their theory of impasses as just described. It also results in a rather impressionistic as well as theoretically cryptic diagram. In the end, Goulding and Goulding failed to delineate either a clear theory or a coherent methodology in their approach to the predicaments of patients with schizophrenia.

The redecision therapy approach in transactional analysis was later revised and enriched by further theoretical considerations and methodological advances from psychodynamic transactional analysis. In particular, with regard to the analytic understanding of schizophrenic pathology, exponents of psychodynamic transactional analysis (Novellino, 1991, 2004a [1998], 2004b; Novellino & Moiso, 1990) described a structural model that supports the idea that fundamental intrapsychic conflicts between primitive somatic-affective ego states lie at the base of the structural organization of psychosis. In the work of these authors, the structural conflicts between ego states refer to the internal dynamics of the Child and are more accurately explained by the presence of second-degree impasses (P_1/C_1) or, in some cases, even better by third-degree impasses (P_0/C_0) that are responsible for developmental arrest or ego fixations and regression of the ego/self (see Figure 3.1).

According to these perspectives, the schizophrenia-like psychotic structure can thus be understood in terms of intrapsychic conflict—derived from internalizations of object relations (Fairbairn, 1952)—between ego states within the *archeopsyche* or Child ego state (C_2).

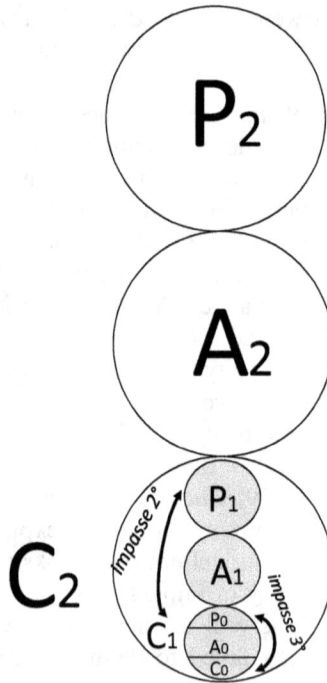

Figure 3.1 The intrapsychic conflict model of schizophrenia (based on Goulding & Goulding, 1979; Mellor 1980; Novellino, 1990, 1991, 2004a [1998], 2004b)

Another fundamental contribution to the understanding and treatment of psychoses undoubtedly remains the work of Schiff (1975) and her colleagues. The Schiffian approach delineated specific communication and psychodynamic aspects of schizophrenia that can be summarized as follows:

- *Symbiosis* as archaic unresolved structural and functional dependency on significant others.
- *Passivity* as a behavioral manifestation of this relational dependency and its perpetuation through discounting.
- The *frame of reference* as a compromise between the intrapsychic and relational worlds as well as a filter with external reality in the absence of real boundaries.
- *Redefinition*, through which the individual maintains his or her frame of reference and carries out his or her life script, which is characterized by unresolved aspects of the original symbiosis.

Despite the attention given by Schiff (1975, Chapter 3) and her colleagues to the processes of exclusion, her structural model of psychosis was developed within a conflict theory of personality. Essentially, she wrote that schizophrenia "is characterized by a locked system of messages in the Parent, corresponding adaptations in the Child, and an Adult which is misinformed" (p. 74). Consequently, the focus of her theory was on the dictatorial role of the Parent (P_2) and the hyperadaptations of the Child (C_2), which leads to pervasive dysfunctional reality testing by the Adult (A_2) of the psychotic patient (through discounting and redefinition).

However, it is here that one of the most significant paradoxes of this model can be found. Specifically, active psychosis is deemed to be, on the one hand, a manifestation of the Child, but on the other, its pathology is treated—both on a structural and a transactional level—as if the Adult and the Child were structured, even during the period of the psychosis, as sufficiently organized egoic systems and subsystems.

In addition, it is of note that the articulate description of various types of schizophrenic psychoses given by Schiff (1975, Chapter 6) reveals the difficulty in further clarifying various aspects of schizophrenic psychosis that are somehow constrained within a model of personality based on intrapsychic conflict and interegoic symbiosis.

In Schiff's approach, the psychopathology of schizophrenia is interpreted according to theoretical conceptualizations (such as frame of reference, double contaminations, transactions of redefinition, etc.) and an old energetic model of the mind and brain that is not consistent with the diverse clinical phenomenology of this disorder or the scientific advancements produced over the last decades in the fields of affective and cognitive neuroscience, infant observation and infant research studies, and psychopharmacological research on psychotic disorders.

More specifically, the Schiffian theory of psychosis does not seem to acknowledge or describe adequately peculiar characteristics of schizophrenic pathology, including:

- The interplay between past relational trauma and primal exclusions.
- The more pervasive existential aspects of ego-self fragmentation and alienation (e.g., the uncertainty of being, the subjective sense of feeling lost, the feeling of losing oneself, emotional withdrawal, etc.).
- The strongly held subjective sense of the absolute certainty of delusions and hallucinations.
- The protocol level of specific psychotic experiences (e.g., visual and tactile hallucinations, passivity phenomena, catatonic states, somatic anxiety, etc.).
- The disruption of personal narrative as manifested by severe thought disorders (e.g., loosening of associations, thought insertion, though withdrawal, thought broadcasting, neologisms, etc.).
- The lack of ego boundaries leading to overexposure to others and the world (intrusiveness from and bodily adhesiveness to others and external reality).
- The more complex transferential and countertransferential enactments that occur, beyond symbiosis, in the here-and-now relationship with individuals with schizophrenia.

A relational, trauma-based model of schizophrenia

The premise for establishing a bipersonal relational perspective to help us understand schizophrenic psychoses requires—in order to remain within a transactional analytical framework—adherence to a principle of human (before intellectual) proximity to the distress of the psychotic individual, without the conditioning that derives from conceptual prejudices. This attitude aligns with the Bernean maxim to "look at the ground first, and then at the map, and not vice versa" (Berne, 1975b [1972], p. 452).

It is actually by exploring the unconfined territory of schizophrenias that one encounters people whose history is often marked by relational traumas, fundamental deficiencies in their emotional diet, and absences and discontinuities in their own experience of being and whose present is pervaded by an existential precariousness, an immediacy—signifying a lack of mediation and filter—in relationships with others and the world. Overwhelmed by ineffable emotions, suddenly depleted of their own thoughts, hallucinating, delusional, jolted out of contingent space and time, psychotic individuals appear to be reaching out with their speaking bodies.

An up-to-date map with which to view the world of schizophrenia must, therefore, not only consider the subjective idiosyncrasies of the schizophrenic experience but also use new lenses through which the analyst/therapist can finally meet the individual with schizophrenia in the first person.

The case of Cary: Berne's legacy regarding splitting in schizophrenia

In his description of the case of Cary in *A layman's guide to psychiatry and psychoanalysis*, Berne (1969 [1957]) described a crucial step in which some clinical manifestations of schizophrenia were not adequately explained by an intrapsychic conflict model of the mind. Here the germ of Berne's splitting model of schizophrenia can be found:

> Cary's mind was split in another way, besides being cut up into separate pieces each acting as though the others didn't exist. The sights which met his eyes and the sounds which came to his ears were split off from his feelings so that the reality did not call forth the normal emotional responses. ... His feelings seemed to have no connection with what went on around him. His mind was split two ways, so to speak, up and down, and also across. These splits remind one of the up-and-down split in the Church during the Middle Ages, which was called the Great Schism, and of how a certain rock called "schist" splits across when it is under stress. The schisms in such frenzied minds is what leads us to call all such conditions "schism phrenesies" or schizophrenias.
>
> (pp. 188–189)

In Cary's case, Berne (1969 [1957]) seemed to envisage the possibility of two different types of pathological dissociation in psychosis, for which he used the verb *split*: vertical splitting and horizontal splitting. Vertical splitting in psychosis can also be seen in individuals affected by various types of dissociative disorders (e.g., dissociative identity disorder and paranoid, schizoid, and borderline personality disorders). These disorders clearly correspond to what previous authors—including Sullivan (1953), Searles (1965 [1959]), Laing (1959), and Berne (1975a [1961]) himself—referred to in the mid-20th century as cases of pseudoneurotic schizophrenia, hysterical schizophrenia, ambulatory schizophrenia, and dissociative schizophrenia. Overall, they described many cases that involved overt switching of identity states—clearly dissociative disorders—that therefore included a broader group of individuals than those who would be generally classified as schizophrenic today.

This vertical splitting involves a type of dissociation that has a particular alternating pattern. It directly relates to splitting in Klein's (1997) sense of bipolarity (good-bad) and Berne's (1975b [1972], p. 134) sense of opposite ego states (Fairy Godmother and Witch Mother). Generally, it involves a dramatic switch or shift in the person's affective state, including experiences of the self and expectations of the other.

Perhaps it is the ability to switch to an alternating self-state, which exists in cases of paranoid schizophrenia, that affords some stability and organization and thus avoids the ego fragmentation found in more severe forms of schizophrenia-like psychoses (e.g., simplex, disorganized or hebephrenic, and catatonic types).

In Berne's view, splitting as a structural feature of schizophrenic pathology is not merely a theoretical construct but refers to real past-life events and relational experiences of the developing individual with historical others. What is pathological in the schizophrenic condition compared with healthy development is the defensive compartmentalization of such experiences within the person's ego.

The more implicit assumption that underlines my own view of splitting as being associated with the structural pathology of schizophrenia is that there is a parallelism between the various types of schizophrenic pathology and ego development. This permits bidirectional influence between relational struggles in early childhood and the structural pathology of the specific type of psychosis.

What seems relevant in this respect is that the ego in paranoid schizophrenias, compared with more severe types of schizophrenia, has reached a more developmentally mature internal organization. As such, vertical splitting would compartmentalize the patient's ego into two main (i.e., opposite) clusters of thoughts, feelings, behaviors, and bodily experiences, each with a semblance of self-consciousness. Moreover, the segregation between two opposite selves in paranoid schizophrenia is never total, but the greater the vertical split of the patient's ego, the more severe the psychosis. In contrast, less differentiated forms of schizophrenia are characterized by less organized ego structures that would, in turn, be more prone to multiple fractures. The fragments in such cases would lack internal coherence and therefore integrity (as will be discussed later in this chapter).

These considerations are also corroborated by initial as well as more recent epidemiological observations that together demonstrate how the paranoid subtype usually has a later age at onset, whereas simplex, disorganized (or hebephrenic), and catatonic subtypes are normally earlier and more insidious in onset (Beratis et al., 1994; Fenton & McGlashan, 1991; Kendler et al., 1984; Perälä, 2013; Sadock et al., 2015).

This vertical splitting was originally described by Janet (1974 [1889]), who theorized that dissociative symptoms were attributable to split-off or dissociated parts of the personality. These psychological structures have their own personal traits, which Janet conceived of as coexisting. These traits think and react simultaneously at a subconscious level but are also capable of taking over consciousness (van der Hart & Friedman, 1989).

On the other hand, Jung (1977 [1908]), who was undoubtedly influenced by Janet's work, compared dissociation to splitting:

> We have taken over from French psychology a similar concept which initially was true for hysteria—namely "dissociation." Today, the name means a "splitting of the self." Hysteria is primarily characterized by dissociation and because dementia praecox also shows splitting ("Spaltung"), the concept of dissociation seems to "run into" the concept of Schizophrenia.
>
> (p. 335)

More interestingly, Janet's (1920 [1907], 1974 [1889], 1977 [1901]) ideas clearly influenced Freud's original work on hysteria when the latter, before developing psychoanalysis, used Janet's ideas on dissociation and embraced Breuer's view of the "double-conscience" (i.e., splitting of consciousness) (Breuer & Freud, 1955 [1895]) as characterizing the hysterical condition. Freud enthusiastically pursued a model based on the belief that hysteria invariably had its origin in historical relational trauma (i.e., sexual abuse occurring in early childhood).

This discussion about the possibility of vertical splitting in psychosis was later resumed by Berne (1975a [1961]) in *Transactional analysis in psychotherapy* when he quoted the first prepsychoanalytic studies of Breuer and Freud (1955 [1895]) in relation to the advanced structural analysis of ego states. In this short but clear passage, he implicitly referred to transactional analysis as a sort of para-Freudian or, if you like, a neo-Janetian clinical approach to the study of human personality, particularly in relation to the formulation of ego states and their mostly preconscious nature together with intrinsic unconscious components that are not necessarily repressed: "For reasons which were particularly cogent at that time, Freud's attention was diverted from structural considerations into the area of psychodynamics, and this eventually resulted in a structural scheme which was conceptual, rather than clinical" (Berne, 1975a [1961], p. 210). Unlike Janet, however, and definitely more in keeping with the psychoanalytic tradition, Berne strongly emphasized the therapeutic worth of the meaning of psychotic experiences and of connecting them back to the personal history and life events of his patients.

Moreover, what Berne further identified in psychosis—as his analysis of Cary's case illustrated—was the copresence of a different form of splitting, which can be called *horizontal splitting*. This conception is close to Fairbairn's view of schizoid phenomena, which clearly influenced Berne's formulation of ego state theory and his advanced analysis of the Parent within the Child ego state (Berne, 1975b [1972]; Blackstone, 1993). Fairbairn (1952) suggested that we must go back to ideas about hysteria (i.e., to dissociative psychopathology rather than to neurotic, superego-based psychodynamics) if we are to understand the schizoid self (i.e., the split ego) and therefore schizophrenia.

Within transactional analysis, a more heuristic description of the schizoid process can be found in the work of Erskine (1993, 2001), Erskine et al. (2001), Little (2001), O'Reilly-Knapp (2001), and Yontef (2001). Horizontal splitting is, in fact, similar to the notion of repression in the sense that some experiential information is not made available to Adult ego state awareness (A_1 or A_2). However, with regard to the structural pathology of schizophrenia, the horizontal splitting described here is essentially distinct from Freudian repression. It keeps unconscious thoughts, emotions, and bodily experiences out of awareness in order to maintain the cohesion of the nuclear ego-self. In other words, this form of splitting is a more basic strategy that the emerging self (C_1) may use to cope with an early, persisting traumatic object, part-object, and/or preoedipal relationship that the person cannot articulate or resolve.

In the face of early relational struggles with reference others, what the developing child cannot articulate in either words or images becomes prematurely dislocated from the symbolic realm and, by means of horizontal splitting, may lie dormant at a bodily-emotional level of experience. It is my view that psychotic breakdown brings to the body's surface what had been horizontally split off from the conscious mind as early as those phases of psychological and neurobiological development (from conception up to 3–4 years of age) when no episodic (i.e., autobiographical) memory is yet available to the developing self. This is, therefore, nonconscious subsymbolic material still in need of a more symbolic organization. What seems peculiar in psychosis is also the subsequent unconscious and preconscious distortion this bodily-emotional material undergoes as a result of the not-yet organized activity of A_1, that is, Berne's Little Professor. This is, in turn, able to produce potentially aberrant experiences of one's self in relation to others and external reality as expressed in certain forms of delusion and hallucinatory phenomena (see "Structural analysis of schizophrenic psychoses" in this chapter).

Overall, in schizophrenia, the peculiar combination of vertical and horizontal splitting within the Child ego state (C_2) is psychodynamically linked to a more pervasive, noncohesive disorder of self-experience that represents a unique type of ego/self-pathology that will be structurally defined in the next section as *Child ego-self fragmentation*.

Primal exclusions and self-fragmentation

Later in *Transactional Analysis in Psychotherapy*, Berne (1975a [1961]) no longer referred exclusively to the concept of splitting but more generally to exclusion. By so doing, he embraced various psychodynamic processes such as splitting, dissociation, denial, isolation, withdrawal, and even repression in order to describe the structural pathology of schizophrenic psychoses and the complex and varied phenomenology of psychotic symptoms.

What I propose here is a review of the structural model of schizophrenic psychoses that, without ignoring Parent/Child contaminations, puts greater emphasis on Parent exclusions at different stages of ego development in order to explore psychotic pathology from a different perspective. Specifically, the Parent exclusion is meant to represent an extended and extremely debilitating deficit in the psychotic structure resulting from early and pre-egoic misattuned and variously traumatic relationships between the developing child and the father and/or mother and/or any other caregivers who played a parental role in the individual's life (P_2–P_1–P_0). This is congruent with what Berne (1975a [1961]) wrote in relation to psychoses: "The situation of the Parent varies and is a strong determinant of the specific form of the psychosis" (p. 139).

Because the subjective drama of the schizophrenic involves primarily the deepest structures of the Child ego state (i.e., the self), a new structural model of schizophrenic psychosis needs to be based on a transactional analysis model of personality that structurally encompasses the self. Such a model is offered by a two-person relational transactional analysis approach as outlined, in particular, by Erskine and Trautmann (1996), Erskine, Moursund, and Trautmann (1999), and, more importantly, Hargaden and Sills (2002, 2003). In particular, Hargaden and Sills used the original structural model of ego states (Berne, 1975a [1961]) as the vehicle for a theory of the self in relational transactional analysis.

According to Hargaden and Sills, the psychodevelopmental roots of the Child appear to be linked in a coherent egoic organization based on a plethora of pre-egoic and fusional states relating to very early periods of development when the individual is not yet able to distinguish an "I" from a "you" and a "me" from an "other-than-me." These preverbal ego states have also been defined as systems of ego/self-activation (Hine, 1997), states of mind (Allen, 2000), and ego/self-states (Hargaden & Sills, 2003), with the subconscious, unconscious, presymbolic, and therefore protomental nature of experiences attributed to the never-ending structural organization of the developing Child ego state. It follows that the structural models originally proposed by Berne (1975a [1961], pp. 48, 55, 63, 145) to explain the clinical symptoms of psychosis, including hallucinatory phenomena (Berne, 1975a [1961], p. 62), should appropriately be extended to the Child ego state/self-structure (C_2) and therefore to P_1, A_1, and C_1 as well as to earlier pre-ego states (P_0, A_0, C_0).

The thesis I present here is based on four intense consecutive years of clinical experience and research with adult patients suffering from schizophrenia-like psychoses, a considerable number of whom were experiencing their first psychotic episode. Despite acknowledging the presence of a variety of psychosocial, genetic, and biologically stress-mediated factors in the pathogenesis of schizophrenic syndromes, a careful analysis of these psychotic patients' personal and psychiatric histories consistently revealed two kinds of fundamental stressful microenvironmental experiences that significantly and chronically characterized their childhood and adolescence.

These two types of traumatic experience can be classified as: (1) experiences of early and enduring abuse (physical, verbal, emotional, and/or sexual abuse that exposed them to various forms of pathological symbiosis); and (2) experiences of early and enduring neglect (abandonment, domestic neglect, homelessness, presence of serious mental and behavioral problems in parents, separation and/or a highly hostile divorce between parents, frequent change of residence, difficult foster care, etc.). Moreover, regardless of the content of the traumatic experience, whether it involved abuse and/or neglect, the type of schizophrenic psychosis is more determined by the timing and degree of traumatic relational experiences between the child and the parents and/or primary caregivers. The earlier and more pervasive the Parent exclusion, the more severe the psychosis.

Structurally, the floridly acute psychotic state can be represented (Figure 3.2) by an excluding, fragmented Child (C_2) where exclusion of the Parent ego state at different stages of psychodevelopment (P_2 and P_1) is present and somatic-affective material coming from the Child within the Child (C_1) is barely available to an emerging reflective Adult (A_1 and A_2) that has, in turn, become prematurely unintegrated, both structurally and functionally, by relational retraumatization.

More specifically, in Figure 3.2, the excluding Child is rendered by a continuous and darker circular line—in comparison with the others—that signifies both the rigid defenses put in place by the Child ego state and the rigidity of its boundaries. This rigidity then exposes the psychotic person's Child to multiple internal scleroses, represented in the figure with both vertical continuous lines—such as the one that divides P_{1+} and P_{1-}—and with horizontal lines—such as the ones that divide P_1 from A_1, and A_1 from C_1. From a psychodynamic point of view, the internal scleroses of the Child ego state corresponds to processes of splitting, vertically and horizontally, respectively, as previously discussed (see section "The case of Cary: Berne's legacy regarding splitting in schizophrenia").

Furthermore, the specific, broken line around the letter "A" illustrates the lack of development and integration of a reflexive Adult ego state from the early stages of life (i.e., A_1 as well as A_2) due to the direct effect of relational and nonrelational traumatic experiences on the psyche of the evolving individual.

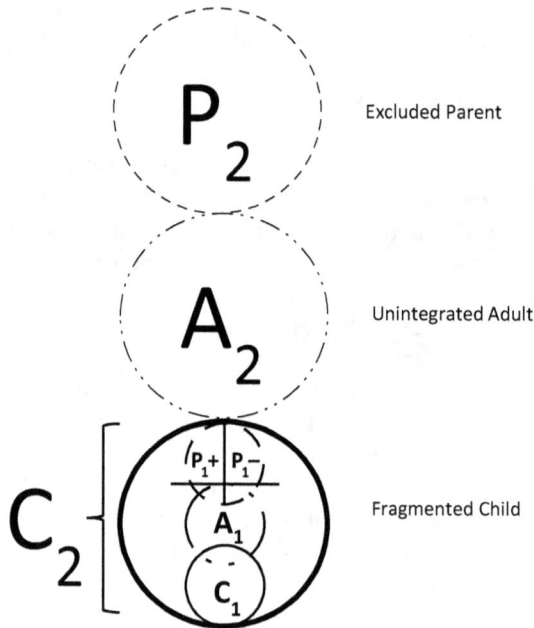

Figure 3.2 The fundamental structure of active schizophrenia

Finally, the circle that indicates the excluded Parent ego state is rendered, according to Berne's original morphology (1975a [1961]), with a dashed line. Indeed, Parent exclusion in schizophrenia is seen here as the endpoint of very early multiple splitting processes affecting the developing ego during childhood and adolescence as a result of traumatic disturbances and discontinuities within the realm of early object relationships between the emerging self and reference others (P_1).

This is in contrast to the more simplistic view of Berne (1975a [1961]) that "not only each neurotic, but each mental defective, each chronic schizophrenic, and each 'immature' psychopath has a well-formed Adult" (p. 59). Instead, attachment studies and clinical research all point to a different view. Early and chronic relational trauma interrupts the capacity to form self-narratives, thus creating rigid divisions and fractures of self-experience that lead to fragmentation of the individual's psyche. This means that assuming a well-formed integrating Adult ego state, as laconically (and rather romantically) purported by the motto "Assume Adult—until proved otherwise" (Tudor & Summers, 2014, p. 60) or, even worse, assuming that we as people "are conceived Adult" (p. 56) is no longer a tenable position in light of recent discoveries and scientific advances in the field of biological research on brain development and their psychotherapeutic implications. More specifically, I am referring here to multimodal in vivo imaging studies of large healthy samples followed over time that are providing relevant information on brain structure (using anatomical magnetic resonance imaging or MRI), axonal connectivity (using diffusion tensor imaging or DTI), brain function and perfusion (using functional magnetic resonance imaging or fMRI), and neuronal density and metabolism (using magnetic resonance spectroscopy or MRS).

Therefore, it is my view, which is more in line with current neuroscientific research and, more interestingly, with Berne's (1975a [1961]) original epigenetic theory of personality, that the Child is the part (structure) with which we are born. And the Child, from conception, comes to exist as an integrating body-ego (A_0) only within an interbodily thread of prelinguistic, sensate, and highly emotional transactions and gestures as well as behavioral and organic (i.e., related to bodily fluids) exchanges between the emerging self (C_0) and a holding and regulatory other (P_0).

Biologically, then, the integrated/integrating Adult does not correspond merely to the development of fully formed (or well-organized) biological structures that persist (also anatomically) over time. It also relates more to rather complex age- and stage-related "experience expectant" and "experience dependent" (Greenough et al., 1987) neurobiological dynamic processes of "sprouting" and "pruning" of connections throughout all brain regions. These processes thus involve the ongoing interplay of genetic and environmental factors, and all together they demonstrate how the development of a normal brain is orderly and follows regular patterns over time (Stiles & Jernigan, 2010).

Most importantly, in line with these more contemporary views stemming from developmental psychology and neuroscience, the specific experiences of the individual with reference others during the early postnatal period, and then throughout childhood and adolescence, seems to play an essential role in establishing the evolving organization of the brain. In referring to these experiences of relational mutuality between the developing child and caring adults, Fisher, Frenkel, Noll, Berry, and Yockelson (2016) coined the phrase *serve and return* interactions: "Children naturally serve when they initiate interaction through gaze, vocalization, and action; adults return the serve when they respond in developmentally supportive ways" (p. 4).

One could thus arguably infer that fragmentation, seen especially in first-episode schizophrenia, corresponds biologically to the progressive, and at times transient, lack of a coherent organization at both an anatomical and a functional level of multiple (also phylogenetically different) brain structures. At a more psychological level, fragmentation may occur as a result of recurrent splitting in place of any other more adaptive defenses, including dissociation (Bromberg, 1998), and when any environmental resources (e.g., access to responsive relationships with caring adults, a secure environment, etc.) cease and/or have never been truly available to the individual early in his or her development and for a prolonged period of time, up to the first psychotic breakdown. Psychosis, then, would eventually coincide with the loss of that fluid plurality of the ego and, therefore, of the person's self-experience, as we know from the functioning of "healthy enough" individuals.

Structural analysis of schizophrenic psychoses

From the point of view of second-order structural analysis, it is possible to distinguish two basic organizations of schizophrenic psychosis: (1) paranoid psychoses; and (2) schizoid psychoses. A useful way to draw the structural diagrams of these is to use Berne's (1975a [1961]) metaphorical definition of exclusion: "the exclusion is like a one-way glass" (p. 66).

Paranoid psychoses

In paranoid schizophrenias, the primarily excluded Parent (P_1), which mainly contains the precipitates of traumatic object relations with one or more parent figures (persecutory, bullying, verbally and/or physically violent, psychologically abusive and therefore symbiotic), looks through a one-way glass down to the Child (C_1) and the Adult (A_1) (Figure 3.3). Through this process, hallucinations (usually auditory and/or visual), persecutory delusions, and ideas of self-reference arise in paranoid schizophrenia (Figure 3.3), although they may also occur in other forms of psychosis (including bipolar disorders).

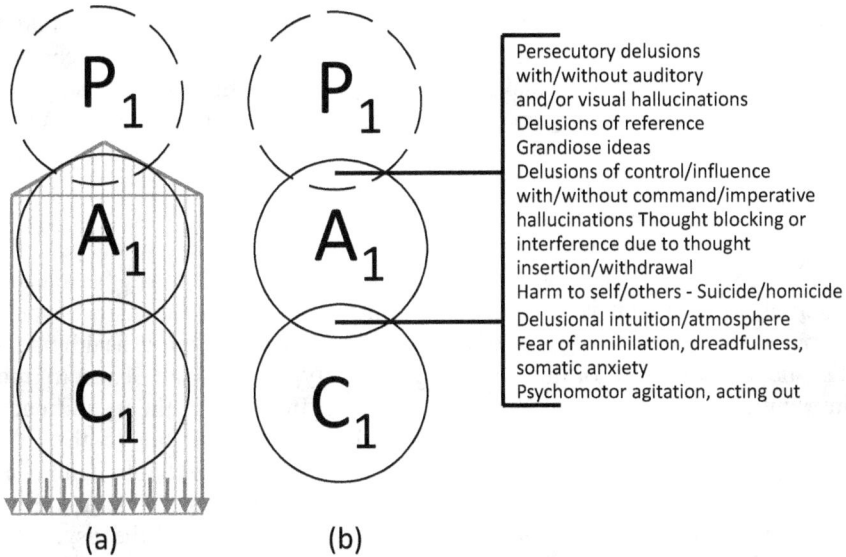

Persecutory delusions
with/without auditory
and/or visual hallucinations
Delusions of reference
Grandiose ideas
Delusions of control/influence
with/without command/imperative
hallucinations Thought blocking or
interference due to thought
insertion/withdrawal
Harm to self/others - Suicide/homicide
Delusional intuition/atmosphere
Fear of annihilation, dreadfulness,
somatic anxiety
Psychomotor agitation, acting out

(a)   (b)

Figure 3.3 (a) Structural diagram of paranoid psychosis (b) Phenomenology of paranoid psychosis as a result of complex exclusions and contaminations of the
Child (pre-)ego states

Figure 3.3 illustrates the intrapsychic experience of the paranoid patient's
Child ego state. The main focus in this figure is on the primary exclusion
process of the Parent, which is represented—again following Berne's diagrams
(1975a [1961])—with a dashed circular line, this time running around the
Parent within the Child ego state (P_1). The effect of the one-way glass produced by the exclusion of the Parent is rendered with a group of darker
arrows pointing downward to indicate the disturbing influence that the Parent
continues to exert on the rest of the emerging self (A_1 and C_1). In addition to
the primary exclusion of the Parent (P_1), the figure shows a concomitant
process of contamination—rendered with an overlap of circles, P_1 on A_1 and
C_1 on A_1—which explains the altered perception that the psychotic self has of
reality and significant others that brings about a range of psychotic experiences that are typical of paranoid schizophrenia (as specifically illustrated in
Figure 3.3b). The primary Adult ego state (A_1) is rendered with a continuous
circular line to denote a greater egoic organization of the Child (C_2) in paranoid schizophrenia compared with what is found in more fragmentary and
undifferentiated forms of psychosis (see also Figure 3.4).

Based on this structural articulation of the inner world of paranoid individuals, their relational world develops around the need to defend themselves
from the threatening gaze and persecutory presence of the Other. The extreme
solution to the anguish of succumbing to the persecutory Other and then

disintegrating translates into an attitude toward the Other that is perpetually suspicious, up until the point when the person with schizophrenia becomes convinced of the Other's malevolence. This represents the paranoid solution on which the delusion of persecution is based. The result is projection onto others of internal object parts (P_1) that are not only unwanted but even unrecognized as belonging to the psychotic person.

Another phenomenological feature (based on subjective experience) of paranoid feeling is a growing pride in the "solitary innocence" of the person's own nuclear self (C_1), which goes hand in hand with hate for the alleged external persecutor. It is relatively common to find a megalomaniacal hypertrophy of the paranoid ego, which blocks the individual from a healthy narcissistic development of his or her personality and instead leads to the involuntary expression of a defective narcissism. In my view, the insufficiency of healthy narcissism suffered by paranoid individuals is due to the self-referentiality of idealized nuclear parts of their own ego (excluding Child) in the absence of a true reflection of the historic Other recognizable as other-than-self (excluded Parent). In this way, the nuclear ego of the psychotic person thickens (C_1) while simultaneously contaminating every possibility of authentic intersubjectivity and intimacy with the primary other (as well as with current significant others).

The fortress of the paranoid ego thus begins to rest on hollow foundations, on "full" voids (i.e., constituent voids of the ego) caused by the "present absence" of the Other (excluded P_1), an Other that one must defend oneself from and stand up to as well as irredeemably sink into.

Schizoid psychoses

In schizoid psychoses (i.e., simplex, disorganized or hebephrenic, and catatonic schizophrenias), the primarily excluded Parent (P_1), which contains precipitates of highly dysfunctional or chaotic relationships with one or both parental figures (physically and/or sexually abusive, mentally disturbed, neglectful, disinterested, incompetent), presents the same situation as a one-way glass but turned upside down. In these cases, the frightened and anguished C_1 searches for the Parent in the presence of a relatively less differentiated and underdeveloped A_1 that has been traumatized by and defensively segregated itself from relatively early and highly dysfunctional object relations (Figure 3.4). This is usually the case with more severe forms of schizophrenia-like psychoses (simplex, disorganized or hebephrenic, catatonic), the phenomenology of which is schematically represented in Figure 3.4b.

In Figure 3.4, the excluded Parent in the Child (P_1)—indicated with the usual dashed circle—is once again the fulcrum around which the inner world of the patient with schizoid psychosis revolves. In the main, this internal world is structured according to a bodily-affective register. This is why the

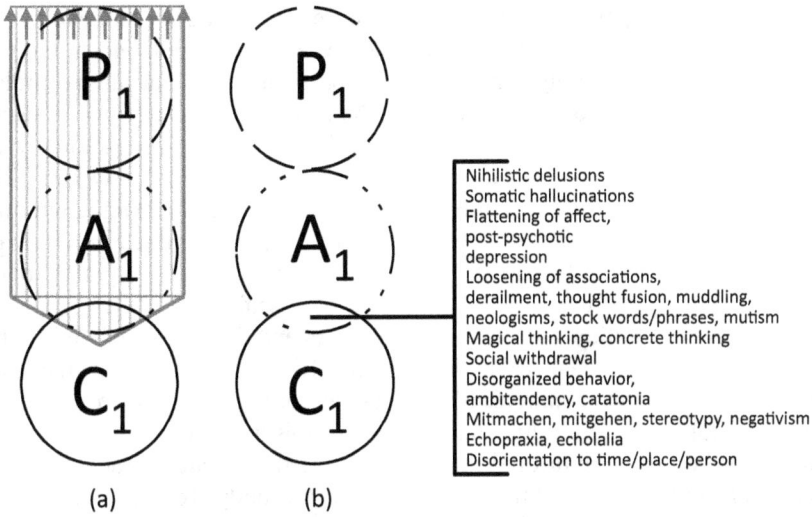

Figure 3.4 (a) Structural diagram of schizoid psychosis (b) Phenomenology of simplex, disorganized, and catatonic schizophrenias as a result of more extensive exclusions of the Child (pre-)ego states in the presence of a weakened/ unintegrated Adult

reader will find, from a structural perspective, a well-defined Somatic Child (C_1) that is essentially the most active proto-egoic structure in this type of schizophrenic psychosis. The upside-down one-way glass effect produced by the exclusion of the Parent is rendered by a group of darker arrows, in this case pointing upward, in order to indicate how abnormal—mainly bodily-affective—experiences in schizoid psychoses (Figure 3.4b) are nonetheless looking for an internal container, a normative and regulatory egoic structure that is still lacking (excluded P_1).

As a result, the development of a reflective primary ego appears to be delayed compared with what one finds in paranoid schizophrenias. This is why the Adult in the Child (A_1) in this figure has been represented with a broken line—different in morphology from the dashed line representing exclusion—that indicates a protomental and intersubjective ego that is still not sufficiently organized or integrated, at the neurobiological level too, due to developmentally unsupportive and chaotic object relations with reference figures.

The term *schizoid* is used here to refer to the main dynamic process that is responsible for these types of psychoses: precisely splitting in its horizontal variant. Indeed, the schizoidism implicated in schizophrenia is essentially different from that found, for instance, in some types of personality disorders, as discussed earlier. Once again, an eminently phenomenological perspective enables us to shed light on the subjective experience of psychotic patients presenting with these other forms of self-disturbance.

Indeed, unlike paranoia, in the experience of psychotic confusion, the Other is essentially indecipherable to the schizophrenic individual. Of the Other the subject can only capture chaotic parts or parts that are psychologically distanced from one another. Thus, the ego in schizoid psychoses begins to find itself in a situation in which it would almost disperse gradually in different directions and toward an unattainable or even absent Other. This process of searching for fragments of the Other leads to the rarefaction and disintegration of the continuous experience of living: the cognitive, emotional, and behavioral life of the ego is at risk of shattering at several points, once again threatening the integrity and identity of the self.

The extreme solution to this psychotic fragmentation is, in this case, the concealment of one's own self in sight of the Other—this is, in fact, the existential meaning of schizophrenic alienation—in the hope that this is the Other who will look for us and ultimately find us. In this way, the person's body, or parts of it, becomes the favored refuge for hiding the psyche, to the point that mental life itself becomes "trans-figured" into the body. To this end, Resnik (2005) talked about "internal projection" (p. 92) of unmentalized or unsymbolized experiences of the psychotic patient into the organs of his or her own body. More recently, Lombardi (2016) described a similar process in his work with psychotic patients in terms of "transference onto one's own body" (p. 49). From this stems the production of bodily experiences and incurable somatic complaints that are aimed simultaneously and constantly at recapturing the attention and love of the Other, which has not yet been completely lost. This alienation of the ego in its own body is, in fact, the prelude to the phenomenological experience of deep loneliness and isolation of the person from the world of external relationships. Bodily introversion seems to be, paradoxically, the only way to avoid depression (a common experience after a psychotic breakdown) and not to die from the traumatic absence of the Other. It is, in fact, an incarnate demand for a relationship with the (new) Other.

Since this withdrawal from the world of object relations is a kind of escape from the ego (or its parts) toward the inside, the hiding place initially offered by the body sooner or later becomes a prison, so much so that the psychotic individual will attempt to evacuate his or her own mind and body somewhere else, that is, into the mind and body of the Other (including the analyst). Psychosis thus results in the sacrifice of one's own ego on the altar of the Other in the attempt to survive psychological death. This evacuation of the psyche from one's own body (mind/body horizontal splitting) to preserve life leads to experiences of disembodiment of the self to the point where psychotic individuals no longer know whether their own mental states—consisting of thoughts, emotions, actions, and even physiological processes in the body—come from their own self or are a consequence of the Other's intervention/interference. Experiences of thought withdrawal or broadcasting, passivity phenomena, and delusions of control are some examples of this process of adhesiveness and intrusiveness of the Other. On the clinical level, these represent the phenomenological features that are distinctive to the schizophrenic experience.

In summary, on the one hand, people with paranoid schizophrenia, who are more prone to vertical splitting, tend to suffer from a form of "bad conscience" by means of which they strenuously preserve a sense of innocence of their own self together with an inflexible suspiciousness toward others, who are invariably perceived as persecutory. On the other, individuals with schizoid psychoses are usually left, as a result of horizontal splitting, with either a mindless body that becomes easily overwhelmed by almost ineffable and disturbing sensory-affective experiences or with a disembodied mind that tends to distance itself from its sensate body while moving elsewhere into someone else's mind and/or body and/or by situating itself in external physical objects or various elements and forces of nature.

In the service of clarity, psychoses have been categorized into two groups mainly in relation to their particular type of trauma-based structural exclusion. In reality, both structural models proposed here can be combined in various ways depending on the psychotic individual's childhood and adolescent experiences. Thus, they can overlap with each other to create particular clinical pictures of psychosis.

In conclusion, at a more structural level, both paranoid and fragmentary psychoses will eventually be influenced and will risk being perpetuated by an Adult ego state—or a "central ego," to use Fairbairn's (1952) terminology—that has been made precarious and unintegrated as a result of relational (re)traumatization. Thus, the ego in psychotic processes is ultimately an ego whose "center cannot hold," to borrow William Butler Yeats's (2008 [1920]) evocative expression.

References

Allen, J. R. (2000). Biology and transactional analysis II: A status report on neurodevelopment. *Transactional Analysis Journal, 30*, 260–269.

Beratis, S., Gabriel, J., & Hoidas, S. (1994). Age at onset in subtypes of schizophrenic disorders. *Schizophrenia Bulletin, 20*, 287–296.

Berne, E. (1969). *A layman's guide to psychiatry and psychoanalysis.* London: Andre Deutsch. (Original work published 1957)

Berne, E. (1975a). *Transactional analysis in psychotherapy: A systematic individual and social psychiatry.* London: Souvenir Press. (Original work published 1961)

Berne, E. (1975b). *What do you say after you say hello? The psychology of human destiny.* London: Corgi. (Original work published 1972)

Blackstone, P. (1993). The dynamic child: Integration of second-order structure, object relations, and self psychology. *Transactional Analysis Journal, 23*, 216–234.

Breuer, J., & Freud, S. (1955). Studies in hysteria. In J. Strachey (Ed. & Trans.), *The standard edition of the complete psychological works of Sigmund Freud* (Vol. 2, pp. 1–335). London: Hogarth Press. (Original work published 1895)

Bromberg, P. M. (1998). *Standing in the spaces: Essays on clinical process, trauma and dissociation.* Hillsdale, NJ: The Analytic Press.

Erskine, R. G. (1993). Inquiry, attunement, and involvement in the psychotherapy of dissociation. *Transactional Analysis Journal*, 23, 184–190.

Erskine, R. G. (2001). The schizoid process. *Transactional Analysis Journal*, 31, 4–6.

Erskine, R. G., & Trautmann, R. L. (1996). Methods of an integrative psychotherapy. *Transactional Analysis Journal*, 26, 316–328.

Erskine, R. G., Hargaden, H., Lynne, J., Little, R., O'Reilly-Knapp, M., Sills, C., & Yontef, G. (2001). Withdrawal, connection, and therapeutic touch: A roundtable on the schizoid process. *Transactional Analysis Journal*, 31, 24–32.

Erskine, R. G., Moursund, J. P., & Trautmann, R. L. (1999). *Beyond empathy: A therapy of contact-in relationship.* New York, NY: Brunner-Routledge.

Fairbairn, W. R. D. (1952). *An object-relations theory of the personality.* New York, NY: Basic Books.

Fenton, W. S., & McGlashan, T. H. (1991). Natural history of schizophrenia subtypes: I. Longitudinal study of paranoid, hebephrenic, and undifferentiated schizophrenia. *Archives of General Psychiatry*, 48, 969–977.

Fisher, P. A., Frenkel, T. I., Noll, L. K., Berry, M., & Yockelson, M. (2016). Promoting healthy child development via a two-generation translational neuroscience framework: The filming interactions to nurture development video coaching program. *Child Development Perspectives*, 10, 251–256.

Goulding, M. M., & Goulding, R. L. (1979). *Changing lives through redecision therapy.* New York, NY: Grove Press.

Goulding, R., & Goulding, M. (1976). Injunctions, decisions, and redecisions. *Transactional Analysis Journal*, 6, 41–48.

Greenough, W. T., Black, J. E., & Wallace, C. S. (1987). Experience and brain development. *Child Development*, 58, 539–559.

Hargaden, H., & Sills, C. (2002). *Transactional analysis: A relational perspective.* Hove: Brunner-Routledge.

Hargaden, H., & Sills, C. (2003). Who am I for you? The child ego state and transferential domain. In H. Hargaden & C. Sills (Eds.), *Ego states* (Key concepts in transactional analysis: Contemporary views) (pp. 185–200). London: Worth Publishing.

Hine, J. (1997). Mind structure and ego states. *Transactional Analysis Journal*, 27, 287–289.

Janet, P. (1920). *The major symptoms of hysteria: Fifteen lectures given in the medical school of Harvard University.* New York, NY: The Macmillan Company. (Original work published 1907)

Janet, P. (1974). *L'automatisme psychologique* [Psychological automatism]. Paris: Félix Alcan. (Original work published 1889)

Janet, P. (1977). *The mental state of hystericals.* Washington, DC: University Publications of America. (Original work published 1901)

Jung, C. G. (1977). On dementia praecox. In *The symbolic life: Miscellaneous writings* (p. 335). London: Routledge & Kegan Paul. (Original work published 1908)

Kendler, K. S., Gruenberg, A. M., & Tsuang, M. T. (1984). Outcome of schizophrenic subtypes defined by four diagnostic systems. *Archives of General Psychiatry*, 41, 149–154.

Klein, M. (1997). Envy and gratitude. In M. Klein (Ed.), *Envy and gratitude and other works, 1946–1963* (pp. 176–235). London: Vintage. (Original work published 1957)

Laing, R. D. (1959). *The divided self: An existential study in sanity and madness.* London: Penguin Books.

Little, R. (2001). Schizoid processes: Working with the defenses of the withdrawn child ego state. *Transactional Analysis Journal*, 31, 33–43.

Lombardi, R. (2016). *Metà prigioniero, metà alato: La dissociazione corpo-mente in psicoanalisi.* Turin: Bollati Boringheri. [Translated into English (trans. unknown): *Body-mind dissociation in psychoanalysis: Development after Bion.* London: Routledge]

Mellor, K. (1980). Impasses: A developmental and structural understanding. *Transactional Analysis Journal*, 10, 213–220.

Novellino, M. (1990). Unconscious communication and interpretation in transactional analysis. *Transactional Analysis Journal*, 20, 168–172.

Novellino, M. (1991). *Psicologia clinica dell'io* [Clinical psychology of the ego]. Rome: Astrolabio.

Novellino, M. (2004a). *Approccio clinico dell'analisi transazionale: Epistemologia, metodologia e psicopatologia clinica* [The clinical approach of transactional analysis: Epistemology, methodology and clinical psychopathology]. Milan: Franco Angeli. (Original work published 1998)

Novellino, M. (2004b). *Psicoanalisi transazionale* [Transactional psychoanalysis]. Milan: Franco Angeli.

Novellino, M., & Moiso, C. (1990). The psychodynamic approach to transactional analysis. *Transactional Analysis Journal*, 20, 187–192.

O'Reilly-Knapp, M. (2001). Between two worlds: The encapsulated self. *Transactional Analysis Journal*, 31, 44–54.

Perälä, J. (2013). *Epidemiology of psychotic disorders.* Tampere: Juvenes Print, Finnish University Print.

Perls, F. S. (1969). *Gestalt therapy verbatim.* Lafayette, CA: Real People Press.

Resnik, S. (2005). *Glacial times: A journey through the world of madness.* New York, NY: Routledge.

Sadock, B. J., Sadock, V. A., & Ruiz, P. (2015). *Kaplan & Sadock's synopsis of psychiatry: Behavioral sciences/clinical psychiatry.* Philadelphia, PA: Wolters Kluwer.

Schiff, J. L. (with Schiff, A. W., Mellor, K., Schiff, E., Schiff, S., Richman, D., Fishman, J., & Momb, D.) (1975). *Cathexis reader: Transactional analysis treatment of psychosis.* New York, NY: Harper & Row.

Searles, H. F. (1965). The effort to drive the other person crazy: An element in the etiology and psychotherapy of schizophrenia. In H. F. Searles, *Collected papers on schizophrenia and related subjects* (pp. 254–283). London: Karnac Books. (Original work published in 1959)

Stiles, J., & Jernigan, T. L. (2010). The basics of brain development. *Neuropsychology Review*, 20, 327–348.

Sullivan, H. S. (1953). *The interpersonal theory of schizophrenia.* New York, NY: Norton.

Tudor, K., & Summers, G. (2014). *Co-creative transactional analysis: Papers, responses, dialogues, and developments.* London: Karnac Books.

van der Hart, O., & Friedman, B. (1989). A reader's guide to Pierre Janet on dissociation: A neglected intellectual heritage. *Dissociation*, 2, 3–16.

Yeats, W. B. (2008). *The collected poems of W. B. Yeats.* London: Wordsworth Poetry Library. (Original work published 1920)

Yontef, G. (2001). Psychotherapy of schizoid process. *Transactional Analysis Journal*, 31, 7–23.

4

FORMS OF TRANSFERENCE AND COUNTERTRANSFERENCE IN ENCOUNTERS WITH SO-CALLED "SCHIZOPHRENICS"

Into the arena: The case of home treatment teams

As a psychiatrist working within a home treatment team in Lambeth in the heart of London from October 2010 to February 2015, I was able to undertake, for the first time and over several years, transactional analysis work with psychotic patients, often at the onset of their schizophrenic pathology and directly in their homes with their families.

Crisis resolution and home treatment teams (abbreviated in the international scientific literature as CRHTs or simply HTs) usually serve adults experiencing an acute mental health crisis who are otherwise likely to require hospital admission. Effective CRHT teams normally include psychiatrists, mental health nurses, support workers, social workers, and clinical psychologists. They aim to provide rapid assessment, looking after patients at home when possible, and to facilitate early discharge from the hospital. In so doing, CRHT teams offer a valid alternative to hospital care by typically providing 24-hour access and a 7-day-a-week home visiting service, gatekeeping functions (i.e., controlling access to inpatient beds and assessing suitability for home treatment before admission), and practical help with daily chores and responsibilities. They provide a high level of clinical and psychosocial intervention and a multidisciplinary as well as an interdisciplinary attitude (Burns et al., 2001; Heath, 2004; Johnson et al., 2008; Wheeler et al., 2015).

The home setting also allowed me to alter the intensity of the analytic setting because I was able to meet the patient more than once a day for individual sessions as well as to meet family members separately and, if appropriate, together with the patient. In most cases, the length of this psychotherapy intervention was the period usually assigned for home treatment, which is about 6–8 weeks duration. During the same period, however, I was able to undertake much longer transactional analysis therapy with psychotic patients from other areas of London outside the borough of Lambeth as part of my part-time private clinical practice, which took place exclusively in the evenings and on weekends.

My continuous work on the home treatment team over those years fundamentally changed my conception of schizophrenic pathology and its treatment, including from a transactional analysis perspective (Mellacqua, 2014). I was able to fully appreciate the truth of Paul Federn's (1953 [1952]) observations on the role of the family and environment in aiding or abetting the analytic treatment of psychotic patients: "Every psychosis is consciously or unconsciously focused on conflicts or frustrations in family life. With psychotics, as with children, the result of a psychoanalysis depends so largely on the helpfulness of the environment" (p. 120).

From these considerations stems Federn's (1953 [1952]) focus on the work of *mental hygiene* with the family of origin and, where possible, with the psychotic patient's most intimate social microgroup (e.g., spouse, partner, children, close friends, colleagues, etc.). At a time when it was believed that no Freudian psychoanalysis was viable for schizophrenia because it is a secondary pathology to primary narcissism, Federn was the first to clearly acknowledge the possibility of a positive transference on the part of the psychotic individual in his or her relationship with the analyst. In this chapter, I address this topic from the theoretical perspective of transactional analysis and suggest, along with what Federn originally acknowledged, that there is the possibility of an anaclitic transference by schizophrenic patients toward their significant others, first and foremost the analyst (see section "From the patient's side", this chapter).

Regardless of the more or less traumatic past of these patients, the anaclitic transference, formed of yearning-for-the-Parent transactions, is based on the conviction of the Child ego state of these individuals that they will one day meet a new Other who will be able to help them make sense of their own experience of confusion, existential loss, or even worse, subjective alienation and fragmentation. This passage by Christopher Bollas (2013) echoes these reflections: "There is not only an unconscious belief in the arrival of this other, but also there will be a search to find such a person, within whose presence those frozen self-states can be released, then conceptualized and, finally, understood" (p. 71).

The following excerpt from a domiciliary session with Paul and his family encapsulates in a few lines the sense of a subjective suffering that longs for relief and the Other's understanding.

(P = Paul, M = Mother, F = Father)

P: (In a trembling voice) I ... I'm not well. I don't feel well... I'm dying (shouting and then crying).

M: I! I! I! And your bloody diseases! You're always saying "I"! What do you want, Paul, from us? (giving a snort of disgust)

F: (Silence)

P: (Addressing both parents): When I say "I" you know I mean "we," I mean that you're there ... right there ... because I live with you, in your house ... I want ...

M: And so stop saying "I"! Stop saying "I want this" and "I want that" ... If we are there... as long as we are there, where are you thinking of going?

P: I want to live!

F: (Silence)

M: And how? By doing drugs with your friends? By going in and out of psychiatric hospitals?

P: Enough! Enough! (putting his hands to his temples) ... Talk to the doctor ... Doctor, you tell them ... I'm ill. They are killing me!

The truth of what Paul says is this: "When I say 'I' you know I mean 'we.'" The suffering of the ego in schizophrenia is thus a suffering that always occurs with the Other, regardless of the material presence of that Other in the patient's actual life. Schizophrenia shows how the Other is primarily the real parent (or a substitute) who has from the earliest periods of development shirked on many occasions, and for a sufficiently long time, the onerous task of facilitating the young person's psychological as well as biological birth. Instead, the person is left prey to an anguish of living, to an unstoppable fear not of death but of the unknown that underpins life itself.

In addition, the Other, because he or she is also an internal Parent—with its intrusiveness and traumatic and toxic inconsistency—becomes part of the patient's ego-body and his or her profound existential pain. Ultimately, the Other, insofar as it is society and the culture of an ethnic group, is also an anonymous Other, therefore potentially ubiquitous, pervasive, and something from which the person cannot escape or become permanently isolated without suffering psychic death.

Schizophrenia teaches us how unexpected existential traumas—especially during periods when our mind is not yet equipped to deal with the level of mental, and sometimes physical, pain associated with them—can also put us in situations that disrupt our still blurred perception of the Other. These traumatic events may include the sudden loss of someone, a physical disability or serious accident, even migration in the context of natural disasters or civil wars. What seems existentially far more traumatizing for the developing individual is the absence or insufficiency of the Other at the time of a traumatic situation, especially if this occurs for prolonged periods during childhood and early adolescence when the person's Parent is not yet psychologically structured or well internalized. This same Parent, from which, unconsciously, we expected unconditional care and love, suddenly becomes— or we ourselves become—fixed in our belief in it, unable to receive that amount of pain itself, to contain and return the pain to us in a form that we find bearable and ultimately acceptable. The pain of the trauma is, therefore, all our own. Indeed, we ourselves are our pain and our incurable disease, and we become lost in a swirl of intense and conflicted questions: "It is not possible!" "No!" we cry.

The pain of the trauma is above all caused by the Other, his or her failures, the fault for which the Other will have to atone until his or her death. But who is the Other? Who are all the others? And so, if this is how it is, "Who am I? To whom does this living thing that I am belong? Whose body is this?" In other words, the person is ultimately left with an image of the Other as a bodily extension of his or her own self, as a physical living body, or a multiplied version of it.

Individuals en route to a pathology such as schizophrenia find themselves encountering two existential extremes: never quite complete adhesion to the Other (through projective identification) or never quite complete alienation (through splitting and body-mind divide) from the Other. In these extremes, the person relinquishes a history of responsibility toward both the self and the Other. Responsibility here means the ongoing ability, including in difficult situations, to know how to react to one's own sensory and bodily experiences, emotions, mental images, thoughts, and behaviors in relation to others and society in general at different stages of development.

The innate paradox in this task of accountability toward the self and others—in circumstances of ontological precariousness and, at times, even physical survival—is that without a substitutional Other right there in the place where we fight our battle for existence, we all risk dying, losing ourselves, going to pieces, and therefore going mad.

The drama of schizophrenic psychosis, therefore, unfolds on at least two basic existential dimensions. On the one hand, processes of primary exclusion initiated by the Child leave the psychotic's self ever in need of a new Parent both at the intrapsychic and the relational level. On the other, exclusion in schizophrenia represents an authentic attempt to rebel against psychological and relational death, to being originally invisible to the Other, so as to set psychic life in motion again where it was interrupted. This rebellion is an attempt to loudly and painfully declare a personal "I" where there is not yet a "we"—in the sense of "I *and* you," "me" and "other-than-me"—in that primitive arena that is always alive and without clear ego boundaries. Berne (1975a [1963], 1975c [1972]) called this area the *primal protocol* or the *tissue level of experience*, where the most intimate emotions in the relationship with the Other (when this Other is not yet perceived by the person as other-than-self) are brought into play, where, without words, we combat hate and love, aggression and abandonment, death and life. Here is a more poignant definition of protocol given by Cornell and Landaiche (2006):

> Protocol is a kernel of nonverbal, somatic experience that may be touched or triggered in intimate relationships. Such moments are often impregnated with both hope and dread. ... Protocol does not

71

exist separate from a person's sense of self but is the very matrix from which we each organize our relational experiences. It is inextricable from our bodies and selves.

(p. 204)

It is for this reason that Paul cries out in anguish, "When I say 'I' you know that I mean 'we.'" It is for this reason that individuals in the grip of psychosis appear to ask incessantly and more or less explicitly, "Who are you really to me?" and therefore "Who am I really to you?" This reminds us, perhaps, of the greatest truth and, at the same time, the most difficult existential task that every human is required to fulfill: the insufficiency of being an "ego" without an Other (or alter-ego) who really wants to be and knows how to be there for us.

The brave analyst

Paul later tried to find a flat where he could live independently. Following this came a series of hospitalizations and returns to his parents' house, living every relapse on the subjective level as if it were a massive failure in his committed attempt to find his "own place" in the world. With every psychotic collapse, he became especially persecutory toward his parents, progressively reducing any social contact until he was completely isolated, spending nearly all his time at home. His favorite hobby became reading books on philosophy and, increasingly, playing video games. With a second period of work with the home treatment team, he was finally able to find himself a supported accommodation and later join a program of gradual integration into employment as a gardener.

I met Paul just after his second hospitalization with the home treatment team in Paddington at a time when he was going through a period of relative mental stability. He had been sent to me for private therapy work. At the time, he had been working as a gardener for about eight months but had cut off all contact with his parents. Our psychotherapy continued for approximately two years, during which time I ensured he had weekly sessions (sometimes three times per week). Throughout the same period, I was able to attend with Paul a series of meetings at the local multidisciplinary community mental health team during which his family doctor, his social worker, his employer, and finally also his parents were present. I certainly do not believe I "cured" Paul's basic way of interpreting other people (primarily his parents) as permanently antagonistic and tirelessly persecutory to his life. I am, however, fairly confident of having enabled Paul to undertake the relatively long and difficult task of individuation. This was made possible not only due to the analytic work we engaged in but also thanks to the multidisciplinary, interdisciplinary effort that enabled him to engage with a diverse group of significant others who were all determined to be "good enough" in their relationships with him. Being good enough in work with patients affected by schizophrenia means bravely inviting them into an intimate "confrontation" of their Child's distressing experiences, encouraging their most authentic aspirations until they can adapt, like everyone else, their own internal images to external reality, including the psychological reality of the Other as other-than-self.

Even more than this, the positive attitude of the therapist in the face of the confrontation is, in Berne's opinion (Berne, 1975c [1972], pp. 305–307), what makes a therapist brave. The bravery required of analysts working with psychotic patients, however, appears to be much more far-reaching than Berne first envisaged. It is less about dealing with psychotic patients at the limits of their tragic life script and more about identifying a greater tragedy—that is, their lack of a well-formed life script that has been substituted for from their earliest years by a fragmented protocol. Despite all this, the brave analyst responsibly pursues the main task of guiding schizophrenic patients along their psychodevelopmental course so that they too can coconstruct, thanks to the analytic work and extra-analytic experiences, an increasingly coherent narrative of the self. This can then be translated into a new personal history and real level of experienced life. In this respect, I find myself agreeing with English (1988) when she suggested that

> the imagination [of a psychotic] roams wildly in a disorganized manner precisely because he or she cannot connect and organize fantasies within the structure offered by a script. However inadequate and scary, a script offers possibilities for contrasting fantasies and reality in small ways rather than in an overwhelming, major way.
>
> (p. 297)

The rather mad risk in a deterministic and monopersonal view of schizophrenic psychopathology lies in believing the psychotic person's reference figures to be irredeemably "guilty" for the patient's psychological and existential disease. In contrast with this way of thinking, Berne (1970) had this to say about parental influence on the psychophysical development of children:

> Parental programming is not the "fault" of parents—since they are only passing on the programming they got from their parents—any more than the physical appearance of their off-spring is their "fault," since they are only passing on the genes they got from their ancestors.
>
> (pp. 180–181)

It follows that a causal model of schizophrenic psychopathology, based on the parents' influence, is somewhat reductionist both from a theoretical perspective (it is now scientifically accepted that there is a multifactorial genesis for psychotic disorders) and on an essentially pragmatic level from the point of view of therapy and prevention. However, this does not lessen the role of parental influence on the formation of personality in early periods of psychological development when individuals do not yet have a sufficiently organized Adult, even though their Child appears to already have a feeling of reality based on intuition, primal images, illusions, and, in more general terms, ineffable bodily-emotional-type experiences that are largely protocol-based (nonconscious).

Therefore, in line with Laing's (1959) view of schizophrenia, I believe it is necessary to move away from talking about "parental fault" and start thinking about responsibility to each other as parents (or caregivers), family members (brothers, sisters, partners, etc.), teachers, and even citizens and political leaders. Indeed, society at large includes sensitive individuals whose psychobiology and (poly)traumatic life events are more likely than those of other people to result in experiences of deep ontological precariousness and existential fragmentation. They too, however, are part of the essential basis of all family, social, and community life in a broader sense.

Although during my clinical experience many, sometimes severely, psychotic patients had polytraumatic histories and came from highly dysfunctional families, when their caregivers were present during acute breakdowns and were then accessible afterward during the psychological therapy, I always considered this to be a help rather than a hindrance. Over the years, I also came to realize that the active recruitment of family members for wider analytic work is not always possible for reasons that varied from case to case (organizational difficulties, unavailability of the patient or caregivers, presence of psychiatric disease in relatives, legal issues, etc.). In other words, healthy work on individuation, when possible, should not preclude consensual work of psychoeducation and, better still, psychotherapy for the patient's family members or caregivers in accordance with the pioneering paper by Federn (1953 [1952]) on the work of mental hygiene carried out within the families of psychotic patients.

For the reasons discussed thus far, not including other purely neurobiological considerations, it is also clear that antipsychotic drugs by themselves are not "good enough" for the treatment of schizophrenia. Even if they help to reduce the psychotic anguish (ranging from paranoia to bodily dissociation) of the patient's Child and to downgrade the delusional and hallucinatory experiences, they certainly do not give the patient a new Parent. It is, instead, the responsibility of the analyst, other mental health professionals, and, more generally, the family, and therefore society in a wider sense, to be that flesh-and-blood Other for the patient. Together they need to be and embody that primary Parent whom individuals with psychosis still need in order to access the nakedness of their own being and to become, in their own turn, courageously and responsibly, a "good-enough individual" (Samuels, 2016, p. 105).

From the patient's side

In line with a relational approach in transactional analysis (Cornell & Hargaden, 2005; Fowlie & Sills, 2011; Hargaden & Sills, 2002; Moiso, 1985), the therapeutic encounter with schizophrenic individuals provides a crucial moment during which their historical trauma may reemerge in the form of transferential and countertransferential enactments. If we maintain the distinction presented earlier between paranoid and schizoid psychoses, we see that there are two corresponding transference modalities in therapeutic relationships with these individuals: projective identification (based on the paranoid resolution of the anguish of fragmentation) and schizoid transference (based on the possibility of a bodily relationship with the Other).

Projective identification

In paranoid schizophrenia, transference to the therapist is actualized primarily through processes that can be defined as *ambivalent projective identification* (or *idealizing-persecutory transference*). This leads the patient to experience the Other, including the therapist, as either a good or a bad Parent.

Unfortunately, in other situations, as a consequence of this transferential process, the patient may act out her or his persecutory selfobject (or multiple persecutory selfobjects) derived from internalizing persecutory object relations and projecting them onto either the self or the therapist. This leads to psychological attack, such as verbally and/or physically aggressive behavior toward self and others.

These phenomenological aspects of schizophrenic psychoses also reflect the impact of relational trauma on attachment style and biological and neurological processes (Nijenhuis, 1999; Perry, 1999; Schore, 2003) that reenact and embody the relational victim/aggressor positions (Howell, 2002; Howell & Blizard, 2009), the abused child/abuser (Stuthridge, 2006), and the adversarial transference (Hargaden & Sills, 2002).

On the other hand, the idealizing counterpart of the process of transference, which leads to the projection of idealized elements—which are excluded—of the person's own ego onto the Other (P_1), is what goes on to fuel the hypertrophic thickening of the paranoid nuclear self (C_1). This stiffening of the boundaries of C_1 can once again be understood as a defense against psychotic fragmentation for which the Other is perceived to be wholly responsible with his or her early persecutory, and therefore violent, love and hate.

In this regard, Bollas (1987) framed projective identification in the analytic setting in these terms:

> This transference position is characterized fundamentally by the evacuation of an element of the self into the object by virtue of

intense anxieties. On the other hand, the projected elements may be valued parts of the self placed in the recipient for safe keeping, a splitting of the ego that allows the good parts of the self to survive the bad parts of the self.

(p. 244)

In fact, clinical work shows how the paranoid subject is very engaged in defense against the persecutory Other as well as in the similarly persecutory attack on the Other, endlessly alternating psychological positions from victim to persecutor and from persecutor to victim.

The paranoid solution

Whether because the Other is idealized or persecuted in turn, either way, the paranoid individual comes to accept that he or she is the preferred object of the Other's vicious attentions. The paranoid person's position of centrality in relation to the omnipresent attentions of the Other/World leads to the subsequent delusional structuring of external threats in the form of persecutory delusions.

Moreover, the vertical split of the Parent-within-the-Child (P_1) between Good-Other and Bad-Other and their simultaneous expulsion from the person's nuclear ego (P_1 exclusions) is the paranoid individual's main solution for confronting the anguish of disintegration as he or she strives to preserve the illusion of the structural "entirety" of his or her own ego. According to this perspective, the paranoid ego expels the Other from within during early periods of its development, and thus the Other is excluded but never completely lost, structurally speaking.

To the somewhat persecutory loss of the Other, paranoid individuals are not able to respond with grief and sadness but instead do so with a violent counterattack (often with tragic consequences for themselves and others) on the Other, a hallucinated Other insofar as it is perceived as omnipresent and omnipotent and on which rest all the Good and Evil in the world. The ubiquitousness of this persecutory Other is explained transactionally by its Parental nature. That is, it is experienced as a primal object, an environment-(M) Other, or World-Other, and precisely P_1 and even P_0 in more structural terms.

The denied grief of the early loss of the Other conceals the deepest suffering of the paranoid experience. Namely, the paranoid person does not access the real "sense of the Other" and simply to survive renounces not only any authentic interaction with the Other but any chance of the integration of his or her own ego.

Schizoid transference

To recall, the schizoid psychoses are developmentally earlier forms of schizophrenic psychosis and somewhat more severe types, like the catatonic schizophrenia, the hebephrenic (or disorganized) schizophrenia, and the simplex schizophrenia, the last being a mildly symptomatic type of schizophrenic psychosis and equivalent to undifferentiated schizophrenia. In these cases there appears to be an absence of transference to the therapist. This is actually a phenomenological marker of the historical relational deficit between the individual and his or her parental figures. This later becomes structural in the personality of psychotic individuals in line with the empty child/uninvolved parent positions described by Stuthridge (2006).

At the same time, the schizoid nature of this type of transference becomes clinically evident in the patient's increasing preoccupation with bodily sensations. This fear-laden somatic-affective state within the patient's Child is thus essentially preverbal and intimately related to an early nonverbal, often traumatic experience of more extensive self-fragmentation and annihilation.

Akin to the process of projective identification (Klein, 1997; Ogden, 1992 [1982]) and transformational transference (Hargaden & Sills, 2002), in schizoid transference the psychotic person seeks to shift his or her bodily discomfort onto another person (i.e., the therapist) or onto another body or object, just as a baby does with the body of the parent, a physical object such as a toy, or an animal.

I later found a resonating concept in Bollas (1987), one that he refers to as *extractive introjection*. In my view, this helps to further our understanding of these nonverbal unconscious dynamics between the patient and the therapist. Indeed, this yearning for the Parent, as it unfolds in schizoid transference, has the same "parasitical" quality Bollas (1987) attributed to extractive introjection. In such instances, the patient "assumes that all that is life-enhancing (including destruction) is inside the analyst, thus inspiring him to live as close to the analyst as possible" (p. 164).

What seems far more interesting from a therapeutic perspective is that this tacit, and yet potent, proximity of the subject to the new Other is what potentially prepares the analytic couple for an unprecedented anaclitic experience. I only briefly mention here the anaclitic dimension of this transference and will say more about it later in this chapter.

In fact, recognizing that there is a part of the self that, despite the psychotic storm, longs for a new objective and object relationship in the here and now with the Other (including the therapist) is what makes treatment of schizophrenic suffering actually possible. This way of seeing into the psychotic's suffering allows a move away from an analytic position that is mainly interpretative (and that tends to be monopersonal, that is, enacted by the therapist on the patient), if not frankly a-interpretative (see, for example, Freud, 1963 [1917]; Jaspers, 1972), toward a cocreative methodology—either bipersonal or cocreated by the patient and the therapist—in which the therapist is required to operate at a bodily-emotional level in synchrony with the primary psycho-developmental needs of the patient.

Hypochondriacal collapse and tissue experiences of the self

Based on the considerations discussed so far, we can say that the Child (C_2) of schizophrenics, without the help of a fully developed Adult and because of the enduring nature of exclusion processes, is paradoxically in search of a Parent that has never been sufficiently internalized, integrated, and developed. The Child has been prematurely and chronically dissociated from the Parent either because of the fear of being destroyed or as a way to protect the core and emerging self (C_0, C_1) from traumatizing abandonment and neglect.

When the Little Professor (A_1), in the presence of an unintegrated A_2, fails in its attempt to reorganize the self-experience while making sense of reality and containing the anxious Child (C_1) by constructing more or less systematized delusions and/or hallucinations, a structural collapse of the entire Child ego state (C_2) will likely follow. I refer to this internal process within the Child as the *hypochondriacal collapse* of the Child/self (Mellacqua, 2014) because of its peculiarly psychosomatic nature.

The term *hypochondriacal*, as it is used here, narrows the psychosomatic spectrum to concentrate on the unshakable anxiety psychotic patients experience about having a serious physical illness that affects their body with life-threatening or identity-threatening implications. People experiencing psychosis often express a series of beliefs and somatic complaints, essentially of a delusional nature, that resemble the psychiatric and invalidating condition of hypochondriasis.

This collapse of the psychotic self is reminiscent of the concepts of *auto-eroticism* (Freud, 1958 [1905]) and *autism* (Bleuler, 1950 [1911]) in psychosis, the former in terms of the protonarcissistic stage of ego development, the latter for the active quality of the ego withdrawal from reality to the inner life, and both for the libidinal and emotional investment in the body. This collapse can also be considered an aspect of what has been called in the transactional analysis literature a sort of *folding* (or *introflection*) of the Child ego in on itself (Erskine, 2010, p. 12; Perls et al., 1951). Such a structural collapse will ultimately lead to the emergence of what Berne (1975c [1972]) called the "tissue level" (p. 111) of human experience and what Woollams and Brown (1978) later defined as the "Somatic Child" (C_1).

Berne's conceptualization of primal protocol and his idea of the tissue level of experience would currently be framed as implicit memory or subsymbolic organization. This has attracted growing attention within contemporary psychoanalysis, cognitive research, and affective neuroscience as well as in body psychotherapy (Anderson, 2008; Bucci, 1997a, 1997b; Ciompi, 1982, 2003; Cornell, 2015; Damasio 1996 [1994], 1999; La Barre, 2001; Lemma, 2015; Mancia, 2007; Panksepp, 1998, 2009; Schore, 2003, 2012).

In particular, Bucci (1997a, 1997b, 2008) theorized that the process of putting sensory, motoric, visceral, and emotional experiences into words requires the connection of both verbal (i.e., words) and nonverbal (i.e., imagery) symbols to sensory-affective and somatic (i.e., subsymbolic) information through what she terms the *referential process*.

Instead, the structural collapse of the Child, as seen in schizophrenia, leads to the disintegration of language (which becomes fragmented), the loosening of associations and incoherent thoughts, deficits in the ability to mentalize bodily-emotional experiences, severe dysregulation of reflective function (Fonagy et al., 2002), and the separation of the symbolic from the subsymbolic (Bucci, 1997a). This introflection of the Child ego into its own body often coincides, at a clinical level, with the manifestation of nihilistic delusions and more invalidating hallucinatory sensations (visual, tactile, gustatory, olfactory hallucinations) that are accompanied by signs of the lack of self/ego boundaries (thought insertion, thought withdrawal, thought broadcasting) leading to more pervasive states of defensive alienation and estrangement from others and the real world.

Thinking back to my first clinical meetings with patients affected by psychosis, I still have vivid memories of their confused faces, their shrunken and sometimes huddled bodies, long silences, and above all, my inability to communicate verbally with them. They seemed distant to me, out of my reach, although I was eager to help them with words to reduce the state of visible anguish into which they had sunk. My frustration during these meetings became increasingly unbearable and I often fell back on topics related to pharmacotherapy, the weather, or sport and then hastily took my leave of them. This went on for a considerable amount of time until I came across the work of psychoanalysts such as Bick and Anzieu and later Resnik and Bollas, to name the most significant authors. In particular, Bick's idea (Bick 1968, 2002 [1986]) of "second skin" and Anzieu's (1989) conception of "envelope" attracted my attention because of their continual references to the body dimension of the therapeutic relationship. This is how it came about that I undertook a more systematic study of unconscious processes, including bodily processes, inherent in the analytic encounter with these patients. In parallel with my reading of these authors, I began to extend the time I dedicated to sessions with my psychotic patients by maintaining almost infinite silences and often uncomfortable positions and then finding myself affected by physical pains, my face flushed, my armpits unusually sweaty, painful spasms in my lumbar region, and prey to images and thoughts that were freely associated with these bodily experiences. At the start, all this occurred without any verbal exchanges between us. With the sole exception of patients suffering from severe forms of paranoid psychosis, for whom the silence increased their suspicion of me, I noticed how most other psychotic patients tolerated my physical presence and even my long silences. I noticed gradually how these patients somehow waited for something else to happen in the room, or that they were certain that something inexplicable was already happening, that even a few words could flow between us in a way that was special and not immediately clear and that there was time and ultimately also the desire to grasp the meaning of these together.

Later on, when I started working more intensively with psychotic patients, Bick's descriptions of *second skin* processes (Bick, 1968, 2002 [1986]) as unconscious mechanisms of defense helped me to understand why and how it was so difficult to engage such patients relationally in a more traditional talking cure. Bick understood the function of the skin as a primary container. The internalization of this containing function, according to Bick, provides the infant with a primitive notion of a body boundary, three dimensionality, compartmentalization, and, concomitantly, a psychic container—or *psychic envelope*, to use Anzieu's (1989) more helpful metaphor. Together, these are considered to be fundamental precursors of projective and introjective mechanisms, as we see in very early object relations between the developing individual and his or her reference others. Parental containment, in line with the ideas proposed by Bick and Anzieu, is what supports the growth of the baby's "psychological skin," but when this containment is faulty (e.g., as a result of repeated relational trauma either in the form of abuse or severe neglect), the baby may resort to "second skin" defenses that are pseudoindependent forms of self-protection in order to prevent disintegration. The infant's precocious development of speech, when he or she uses the sound of his or her own voice for self-soothing, or a muscular tension that leads to the body being held rigidly together during periods of stress, are examples of second-skin defensive patterns.

In more transactional analysis terms, examples of primitive psychosomatic solutions to underlying anguish in the psychotic self can be seen in catatonic patients as manifestations of a "frozen Child." As for infants, these psychosomatic enactments may include rigid muscularity and bodily stiffening, a fixed gaze that latches on to something inanimate as a way to hold the self together, holding the breath or closing down the senses, and precocious talking as a way of self-soothing. This all occurs as if the Little Professor (A_1), which had become prematurely lost in verbal transactions, had to let the Somatic Child (C_1) reinvent a bodily narrative of the self-experience.

In fact, psychotic individuals often overuse sensory-affective experience and physical sensation as a way of dealing with their defective capacity for real object relations (P_1 and P_0 exclusions). Psychotic withdrawal accompanied by increased preoccupation with bodily functions paradoxically constitutes a form of medication for the emerging ego that was damaged by early relational trauma and that is incapable of working with real reparative processes.

An extreme experience of relational deficit is often followed by an attempt to fill the empty spaces. In such situations, psychotropic substances (cannabis, amphetamines, cocaine, heroin, etc.), alcohol, and even pseudoactive social involvement in militant unions or religious communities that exert strong Parental roles (with a variety of cultural implications) can form part of the missing P_0, P_1, and P_2 functions. This reflects the strenuous attempt of the emerging self (C_0 and C_1) to construct and maintain a self-identity by looking for the excluded Parent in the real world.

In the context of therapy, the use of a "second skin" (Bick, 1968, 2002 [1986]) by the psychotic individual appears in the form of somatic (body-to-body) transactions with the therapist. This somatic transference is similar to what Meltzer (1975) and Tustin (1990) described in their work with autistic subjects as *adhesive identification*, or to what Resnik (2005) referred to as *bodily identification* in psychosis. In these types of transactions, which occur mostly at a nonconscious level of interaction (Cornell & Landaiche, 2008), both patient and therapist actively participate with their bodily ego (C_1-to-C_1 transactions). The reality of these deep somatic transferences and countertransferences in the therapeutic relationship has forced transactional analysis clinicians to revise TA methodology with psychotic patients in significant areas, particularly those related to "primal images" (Berne, 1975b [1961], p. 208; 1955/1977, Chapter 4) and "primal protocol" (Berne, 1975a [1963], pp. 218–219, p. 228; 1972/1975c, p. 123). As Bloom (2006) proposed, "It could be suggested that in some cases these long held and deeply embedded second skin processes represent an unconscious narrative of their own which run parallel to a more usual psychoanalytic exploration of mental thoughts and images" (p. 59).

In other words, working with psychotic patients reminds us of the considerable importance transactional analysts need to attach to unconscious-to-unconscious communication, which includes both the therapist's and the patient's bodily experiences. Indeed, my clinical work with patients suffering from active schizophrenia has shown me how the unconscious is not only a language but first and foremost bodily grasping and sensate knowing of one's self and others.

In this regard, together with the notion of the primal protocol envisaged by Berne (1975b [1961], 1977 [1955]), I initially found the idea of the *unthought known* developed by Bollas (1987) to be an extremely illuminating concept that helped me, including methodologically, keep the focus on a much deeper level of mutuality, especially with psychotic patients. In Bollas's view, the unthought known refers to what we "know" at some level but cannot express, at least at first, in words. Why such knowledge cannot be verbally articulated emerges from his understanding of how selfhood is formed through otherness:

> The concept of the self should refer to the positions or points of view from which and through which we sense, feel, observe, and reflect on distinct and separate experiences in our being. One crucial point of view comes through the other who experiences us.
>
> (pp. 9–10)

Bollas (1987) also asserted that the shaping of one's subjectivity remains lodged in object relations established prior to the development of thought or language: "The experience of the object precedes the knowing of it" (p. 39). This noncognitive experience of being held by and transformed through the

Other constitutes, according to Bollas, a form of "object-seeking that recurrently enacts a pre-verbal ego memory" (p. 16).

Like Bollas from his analytic perspective, Schore (2001), a researcher in cognitive and affective neuroscience, conceived this nonlinguistic mutuality in terms of a "preverbal bodily based dialogue" (p. 67).

However, it was through my subsequent reading of Cornell (Cornell, 2008a, 2008b, 2015; Cornell & Landaiche, 2006) that I became most fascinated by the body's physicality and its disturbing as well as informative role in the analytic process. For Cornell (2015), the therapeutic process itself "becomes a kind of psychosomatic partnership that can often be wordless, entering realms of experience that may not easily come into the comfort and familiarity of language" (p. 44). His reflections on somatic experiences in the analytic process have proved to be of paramount importance to me as I have become progressively more involved in my clinical work with the most disturbed psychotic patients. Indeed, the challenge of this and the following chapters is to invite a reconsideration of how, with an adequate advance of Berne's theory and methodology, transactional analysts can begin learning how to be receptive to their own somatic and countertransference responses, especially in analytic work with people suffering from psychosis.

Moreover, in my view, transactional analysis can, in turn, contribute a deeper understanding of intrapsychic processes and object relations to the field of both psychoanalysis and body psychotherapy by providing them with a powerfully evocative vocabulary, intuitive diagrams, and more tangible metaphors. As such, it might potentially foster integration between various therapeutic approaches to the comprehension and treatment of schizophrenic predicaments.

From the therapist's side

In general, in every therapeutic relationship, transference dynamics enacted by the patient are associated with similar countertransference dynamics coming from the analyst (Racker, 1957). This is what Winnicott (1975) defined as *objective countertransference* and Clarkson (1992) better expressed as *reactive countertransference* that aims "to emphasise that the psychotherapist is reacting accurately or objectively to the client's projections, personality, and behaviour in the psychotherapeutic relationship" (p. 155).

This is evident in work with psychotic individuals when the therapist is immediately introduced into a relational arena that is densely packed with symbolism, images, allusions, metaphors, and a bodily-emotional (and therefore protomental) narrative in which thoughts and emotions are concrete as well as fragile and labile. These might include small gestures in which a fleeting facial expression or changing inflections in the tone and rhythm of the voice—even the type of clothing worn, body posture, and inanimate objects distributed around the therapy room—all become an intimate part of the analytic setting.

Indeed, as analysts of individuals experiencing a psychotic breakdown, we invariably become immersed in a dense array of subsymbolic experiences that are primarily expressed through an imaginative and bodily register. Therefore, to be able to define the types of countertransference that emerge in the therapeutic relationship with the psychotic person, the analyst's subconscious and unconscious reactions and receptivity to the patient's transference need to be more fully clarified.

For example, during my early work with the most disturbed psychotic individuals, I found myself progressively more aware of my strong tendency to silence the long silences in the room either by saying something to the patient or shifting my attention to extra-analytic concerns and rather often by trying to ignore the growing discomfort in my own body. I was not able to provide my patients, at least initially, with any effective talking cure for their ineffable suffering. Sadly, I was not even listening to them.

I turned to a psychoanalytically oriented transactional analyst for regular supervision, which was deepened by interest in the psychoanalytic works of Paul Federn, Wilfred Bion, and Donald Winnicott as well as more contemporary authors such as Paul Williams, Salomon Resnik, Antonino Ferro, Riccardo Lombardi, Christopher Bollas, and William Cornell. I also renewed my reading of Berne's first writings on intuition and primal images and his germinal ideas about the script protocol in order to address the issues that were emerging in my clinical work with psychotic patients.

For me as young transactional analysis practitioner, this was one of the most exciting and enriching learning periods of my professional life. The repeated experiences of bodily discomfort in the presence of my psychotic patients slowly allowed me to enter a new realm of therapeutic relatedness. Fundamentally, I was learning for the first time as a psychotherapist how to welcome my own somatic experiences into the analytic process without first saying or doing anything. Surprisingly, my psychotic patients would naturally do the same. They would not ask for verbal transactions. If they did, it was more than a request. For example, with paranoid individuals, it was, rather, a more or less explicit invitation to fight, flight, or freeze, whereas with more withdrawn psychotic subjects it seemed at times like a need to be somehow "fed" through my words. Essentially, their bodies and gestures were impacting my unconscious psyche through my bodily senses, making me progressively more aware and disturbed at the same time through my own unlanguaged somatic reactions. Subsequently, images and dreams would come repeatedly, and often rather savagely, to my mind, exposing my own unconscious on the surface of consciousness whether at night, in the middle of a therapy session, or during a bus ride to and from work. A more coherent narrative would come, however, much later in the analytic journey, and not without the help of supervision. Meaning would usually follow after a recurring mutual sharing of complex sensations, bodily-emotional experiences, metaphors, sensate (often silent) interpretations, dream analysis, and progressively more symbolic connections among various situations presenting within and without the therapeutic setting.

More specifically with regard to the transactional analysis of schizophrenic psychoses, the following section relates the unfolding of different levels of understanding of such a "chaotic situation" as Berne (1975c [1972], p. 392) himself more generally defined the essence of transference when it becomes dynamically informed and shaped by the analyst's protocol experiences and countertransference reactions.

Projective counteridentification

With psychotic patients, we are often confronted by the fundamental dilemma of good and bad, salvation and perdition, and death and life as well as, even more critically, the impossibility of choosing between this or that.

This impossibility is not only to be accepted as a given but has deep historical roots for those patients who have in their past actually experienced how love and hate—even when extreme, distorted, and repeatedly traumatic as in the case of Mr Blake (see "Clinical cases," this chapter)—can inexplicably come from the same primary caregiver in circumstances that were unavoidable for the patient because they were experienced during very early psychodevelopmental periods.

Whether as patients or therapists, the entrance into the world of paranoid psychosis seems to confront us with these insuperable polarities of existence and psychobiographical history (a history that may potentially concern the humanity of each of us). In particular, as therapists of psychotic patients, we become, by embodying them, the good Other and the bad Other, the Loved and the Hated, at the same time—and hardly ever, and if so never for very long, one or the other. One is always both of these existences, experienced as an indivisible apposition of contrasting identities or "pieces" of identity that are alien to each other. In certain cases, these are even elevated to the level of magical entities or spiritual beings that are antagonistic toward each other ("You are my angel" or "You are the devil, you must die!") or misidentified as individuals who allegedly and wickedly act on behalf of someone or something else (e.g., an international spy ring, a mafia group, a nefarious organization of pseudomental health professionals, the police, a family conspiracy, etc.).

This is the "pathological ambivalence" that Bleuler (1950 [1911]) wrote of so expertly when referring to the schizophrenic way of feeling and thinking: "a result of conflicting feelings or thoughts flowing side by side, without influencing each other" (pp. 354–355). He subsequently added:

> Even for the healthy everything has its two sides. The rose has its thorns. But in ninety-nine out of a hundred instances, the normal person compares the two aspects, subtracts the negative from the

positive values. He appreciates the rose despite its thorns. The schizophrenic, with his weakened associative linkings, does not necessarily bring the different aspects of a problem together. He loves the rose because of its beauty and hates it because of its thorns.

(pp. 374–375)

The transferential projections—simultaneously positive and negative—to which the psychotic patient subjects us show us those aspects of his or her interior world, a world that also becomes ours and that is not immediately comprehensible. They also exacerbate, while distorting, the inconsistency and perplexity linked to emotional and cognitive experiences that are often irreconcilable among themselves and that, therefore, though pitched at a less intense and explosive level, also color the intersubjective life of those who are supposedly "healthy."

Projective identification can thus be understood at its essence only when one acknowledges its origin and the bipersonal contribution that it makes—namely, that of a primitive, bodily-emotional interaction between the subject (or patient) and its primary object (or significant other).

Moreover, it is worth remembering that Melanie Klein (1997) considered projective identification to be a form of splitting and described how this can be deduced from the two-tone emotionality of countertransference, leading the therapist to face dichotomous counterprojective experiences and behaviors, that is, "white or black" in tone and "all or nothing" in intensity. Consequently, a dichotomy (hate-love, good-evil, persecution-idealization) in the patient's emotional feeling contrasts with a surge of emotions that are similarly dichotomous, irreconcilable, and therefore intolerable. The analyst tries, in turn, to free himself or herself—in the same way the patient does—by expelling them outward. For these reasons, countertransference itself in projective identifications—*projective counteridentification* (Grinberg, 1979)—acquires connotations of both splitting and being alien. These are experienced by the analyst as an attack on his or her integrity or as a morbid paralysis, a sort of mental infection coming from outside that has managed to penetrate his or her mind and threatens to spread systemically and contaminate his or her ego.

It is also as a result of these latter aspects that the concept of projective identification was originally identified by Klein (1997) as an intrapsychic defense and later extended by Bion (1984 [1967], 1977 [1962]), Grotstein (1981, 2005), and Ogden (1992 [1982])—to name but a few well-known authors in this field—as a bridge between the internal and the interpersonal world of both the patient and the analyst.

Projective counteridentification may finally lead, after more or less and often extenuated work with the paranoid person, to a condition of progressive affective estrangement. As a result of this, the therapist may risk distancing himself or herself defensively from the therapeutic relationship, often rationalizing—as happens when using the scalpel of unilateral interpreta-tion—his or her own experiences and those of the patient, thereby inhabiting rather anxiously the role of the "expert" and simultaneously the "controller" of his or her own, the patient's, and others' safety.

Aggressive-paralyzing countertransference

If the relationship with psychotic patients during a phase of acute breakdown and in specific situations (e.g., in a therapeutic setting within psychiatric hos-pitals or prison institutions) starts to show cracks, this can endanger not only the patient's, but sometimes also the therapist's, psychological and even phy-sical integrity.

The dynamics of aggression toward the self and others that can unfortu-nately arise in certain situations in the relationship with psychotic indivi-duals—often complicated by a contextual use or abuse of drugs and/or alcohol—are the result of a deeper process of progressive objectification of the Other (whether a partner, family member, social or health care worker, the therapist himself or herself). Objectification here means flattening the Other to the level of a disanimated object, depersonalizing or dehumanizing the Other to the extent of reducing him or her to a sort of foreign body. As such, it then has the ability to act like an obstacle blocking the way from the inside to the outside, a worrying tumor, a sort of supernumerary aspect of one's self that violently demands the patient's attention. It becomes like a quasi-appen-dix—or better still, a hernia of the intrapsychic world—that irredeemably protrudes toward the outside while remaining irreducible. As such, it is sus-ceptible to hate, negation, concealment, even amputation, because it is instantly considered to be insidious, sinister, and threatening to one's own life.

It is even possible to see the schizophrenic patient's aggression from a pro-tonarcissistic point of view, according to which the patient treats the analyst as if he or she were an extension of the patient's own self (Spotnitz, 1985). The psychotic individual may come to hate and (even physically) attack the therapist in the same way and for the same reasons that lead him or her to hate and want to attack uncontrollably a split and simultaneously negated part of himself or herself. Seen from the perspective of identification and projective counteridentification, the relational dynamics between therapist and schizophrenic patient become the result of a dispersion and simultaneous fusion of the boundaries of each person's ego (even down to experiences of psychic and somatic influencing such as those observed in more severe forms of psychosis as discussed in the next section). In the specific case of aggres-sive-controlling countertransference, the therapist may, therefore, come to feel—especially if he or she has long experience working with psychotic indi-viduals and often with the help of supervision—the same level and kind of aggression and emotional violence toward himself or herself and others from which the patient is suffering.

Schizoid countertransference

A session with a patient in psychosis does not necessarily culminate in identifying and counteridentifying dynamics or in manifestations of marked aggression with potentially dangerous behavior toward both the patient and the therapist. In fact, there are countless clinical situations in which individuals with schizophrenia appear so absorbed in their inner world that they completely, or almost completely, lose awareness of the analyst as a separate object or "other-than-self." This process of apparent withdrawal from the surrounding world—mistakenly thought by Freud (1963 [1917]) to be an absence of transference—instead of distancing the patient from the therapist actually ends up powerfully attracting the analyst to the patient's inner world. Indications of this attraction occur simultaneously in the patient with the loosening—to the point of complete permeability and thus loss—of the boundaries of his or her own ego. On the other hand, the therapist becomes increasingly, and against his or her will, part of the ego-body of the patient and, like the patient, become a speaking body himself or herself.

In such situations, the meeting room—and similarly, the therapeutic setting itself—becomes filled with long, almost intolerable silences. The few words pronounced by either the patient or the analyst remain suspended between long pauses, while the analyst still tries to establish a verbal connection with the patient. Often such an attempt at verbal dialogue will, instead, take the therapeutic couple somewhere else, a place where both the patient and the analyst surprisingly find themselves increasingly absorbed in a different dialectic. This is a nonverbal, sensory, and viscerally mediated unconscious communication that is typically structured as an interbodily narrative, the special semiotics of which are grounded in breathing, subtle features of posture, muscular tension, tone as well as volume and rhythm of the voice, gestures, and even the use made of clothing and appearance (including hairstyle or hair color, beard, tattoos, etc.) during the same session and between one session and another.

In particular, the loss of ego boundaries—or the near lack of differentiation between self and other-than-self—translates into a rising anguish of egoic disintegration for the patient. This is why the patient appears to pay scant attention to the analyst as well as to every other object or phenomenon present in the room intended for the meeting. In reality, even in a state of apparently total estrangement from external reality or in situations in which the patient seems somehow absorbed in a world of hallucinatory experiences, there still seems to be an infantile Child ego state (C_1 and C_0) begging for sensate recognition and relational (even playful) engagement from the Other (the analyst, primarily). In other words, these patients adhere to the therapist with the nakedness of their psyche, which has now become flesh and blood precisely because of the process of introversion that brings to the surface a more nuclear part of their own ego, to which Berne

(1975b [1961]) gave the name "the Child within the Child" (C₁). This Somatic Child (Woollams & Brown, 1978) will be able to employ a sub-symbolic register, rich in polysensory experiences, and use the body as a concrete medium for protomental contact with the Other. In more general terms, one could say that if for these paranoid individuals their anguish is for the Other, for dissociated and alienated schizophrenics, their anguish becomes for their own body, a body that irredeemably bears—from the beginnings of their own life—traces of the Other.

In parallel with the patient's process of introversion, the therapist also experiences a progressive turning inward, thereby exposing his or her own preverbal and bodily self. In this way, the analyst experiences the intrusion into his or her own field of consciousness of nonimages, as well as non-thoughts, together with an array of emotional states of anguish that are, in their turn, disconnected from other unexpected bodily sensations, at times intense, at times delayed, almost always unconscious, and not always imme-diately translatable into words. These are lacunae or fractures in the con-tinuity of the subjective experience of the analyst's ego that catch him or her unaware, as if an internal earthquake had shaken his or her body-psyche in all its conscious and unconscious thickness.

Therapeutic work with even more disorganized schizophrenic patients, often in a particularly acute setting such as the hospital, carries a trace of (inter)subjective experiences of nonrelationship with the historical Other that translate clinically as absences and relational voids in the present analytic arena. In these cases, on the phenomenological level, the analyst often finds himself or herself immersed in a frigid silence with the patient. Later on, and intermittently, he or she may be assailed during the analytic work by crude thoughts and emotions, sometimes associated with fantasies of physical abuse and/or perverse sexual fantasies (including intrusive images while awake and in dreams), recurrent fears of potential physical aggression (in certain cases resulting later in acts experienced for real), up to more or less disturbing experiences of depersonalization, derealization, and fragmentation of the ego. Because of the preverbal and nonconscious nature of these experiences, the therapist is almost never able to distinguish during the therapeutic process which fragmented and dissociated aspects belong to his or her own personal history and which belong to that of the patient.

As in projective counteridentification, the immediacy and unexpectedness of such a vast repertoire of preverbal experiences inevitably leads the therapist to become increasingly aware of these fragmented and dissociated bodily-emotional states within himself or herself—mirroring the process that is hap-pening in the mind and body of the patient—only after having enacted them mentally and relationally and only after having expressed them symbolically, often through an initial register of images rather than words, with the help of regular supervision, and through engaging in a tireless interbodily relationship in the clinical work with these patients.

Anaclitic countertransference

Anaclitic countertransference is the therapist's direct response to transactions in search of a new primary Parent (P_1) originating from the psychotic patient. The distinctive character of anaclitic countertransference lies precisely in its ability to meet, in the here and now, the psychotic patient's psychodevelopmental needs, enabling him or her to reunite the phenomenal (bodily-emotional, cognitive, and relational) and phenomenological (ontological and existential) dimensions within a joint maturative process that we refer to as *personal growth*.

The dynamics of anaclitic transference-countertransference in work with psychotic patients—especially in situations of nascent psychosis and in subsequent conditions of the clinical onset of symptoms—often lead the analytic couple back to early stages of parent-child interaction (although obviously with less archaic ways of interacting) and are entirely centered on the patient's primary needs or hungers (in the Bernean psychobiological sense). These definitely include the need for recognition, for contact, for relief or comfort from pain (both mental and bodily), for nutrition, for protection, and last but not least, for intimacy.

Most likely, recognition hunger (Berne, 1975c [1972]) constitutes one of the epistemological axes of the Bernean transactional theory of human relationships. The evidence for this lies in the fact that every transaction, regardless of the quality and the level of awareness of the ego states of the individuals involved, inevitably entails some kind of recognition of the other (see Chapter 1). That this recognition hunger—in this case understood as recognition of the other as "other-than-self" with his or her own individuality, being taken as given, and being present in the world—was early and chronically disregarded, deferred, diverted, and corrupted can be intuited through the lack of gaze or a gaze that is directed elsewhere (e.g., aimed in front of or inside the schizophrenic patient), often right from the first meeting.

Anyone who has a psychotic patient in analysis hardly ever gives up referring to him or her by name—and does so many times during a meeting, as if the person's name encapsulates a primary need to feed the hunger of the person for being seen, given attention, and recognized as unique. Similarly powerful is the greeting stimulus when encountering the patient even casually outside the therapeutic setting (on the ward, in the street, etc.), as if that patient, on meeting us, is timidly asking for that quick recognition, often returning the greeting with an unexpected gesture, a silent but protracted look, a grimace, an innocent smile, or even an expletive.

Physical contact is another invitation by the patient in psychosis to the therapist. Clinical experience shows how a handshake, a hug, even the patient's request simply concerning how clinical interventions or medical procedures are carried out on the body (e.g., auscultation of the thorax, measuring blood pressure, palpation of the stomach, urogenital examination, etc.) can substitute in some cases for spoken dialogue and induce the therapist to make contact, using his or her own body, with the patient's body. Even aggression aimed at others, when not intent on the annihilation of the other, can be seen similarly according to a psychodevelopmental perspective based on relational needs and particularly on the hunger for physical contact with the Other. As already demonstrated, the psychobiography of severely schizophrenic patients often documents, on the one hand, more or less repeated deprivation of good-enough parental care mediated by physical contact and, on the other, traumatic experiences that have taken a mental form through the traces left (sometimes still visible to the naked eye) on the patient's body (from physical maltreatment to sexual abuse). Physical contact with the therapist can, therefore, both reactivate painful bodily experiences in the patient that have left a distinctive sign even on the psychotic individual's self-image, thereby deforming it, and be, instead, the somatic medium that informs the therapist about the primary needs of the patient, needs that ask to be satisfied through new preobject and object relationships.

The therapist's anaclitic countertransference can also unfold in terms of relational dynamics aimed at guaranteeing relief from the pain that the individual in schizophrenic psychosis is suffering. The nuclear pain of the schizophrenic is an anonymous pain, similar to visceral pain, a deep and dull pain. It is a pain of living that, even when acute, maintains the "object void" to the point of becoming existential anguish. The "void of the Other" left by the exclusion of the historical parent figure(s) leads to the emptying of the person's own ego. Structurally, from a transactional analysis perspective, this process of Parent exclusion will affect primarily the internal coherence and organization of the Child self. This progressive erosion of the Parent within the Child (P_1 and P_0) is the premise for the subsequent leak of the patient's deepest sense of self outside its primitive ego boundaries. In other words, the repeated primal exclusions of the Parent will ultimately be responsible for the "denudation" of the patient's nuclear self. Such a nude self (C_1 and C_0), without the containing and sustaining function of the Parent, either alienates itself in its own body—a process referred to earlier as the hypochondriacal collapse of the Child—or finds refuge and respite in the body-ego of a new Other.

The self in schizophrenia, therefore, moves Other-wards (i.e., toward a new Other), toward a new life, as Resnik (2005) brilliantly explained, boldly making use of the etymology of the word "psychosis," which "comes from the Greek *psyche*, meaning 'spirit, breath of life' and *osis*, animation. It therefore means animating, setting life in motion" (p. 24).

In acute conditions—for example, when confronted with a paranoid individual who is cowering from the fear of being pursued by the mafia or the police, or with a fragmented patient who is in despair because she is convinced she has been raped during the night by doctors, or with an agitated patient stuck in a word salad—the therapist's impulse is to calm the anguish, remove its intensity, almost automatically using caregiving behavior, expressing himself or herself with simple vocabulary and a warm tone of voice, altering its timbre, volume, and rhythm to almost mimic maternal language or *motherese* (Fernald, 1984) in response to a psychotic suffering that has alienated itself even in its language. In this regard, Lacan (1998 [1972]) lucidly clarified how, in active psychosis, the patient does not speak but is noticeably spoken by language to the point of reproducing *Lalangue*, a neologism used by Lacan to meaningfully denote a primitive form of spoken language that involves the lallation of the *infans* (i.e., those who have not yet had full access to the symbolic structure of the word).

The need to be "fed" is also linked to the theme of language. In clinical practice, one may encounter (although rarely in outpatient clinics or private practice) mute patients who adhere to aberrant eating behaviors with dietary restrictions often fueled by delusions of poisoning or ideas of persecution that irredeemably involve the theme of food (see the section "Abena" later in this chapter). In these situations, which are similarly full of anguish and also put the subject physically at risk, it is usually all but impossible to hold back the impulse as a health care professional to feed the patient. This can sometimes lead to strategies such as obtaining sealed food and drink to reassure the patient it is "safe," to, in extreme cases, employing parenteral nutrition or hospital admission for a nasogastric tube.

It is equally the case that the therapist has a similarly impelling desire to talk to the patient as a way of feeding him or her, even if the food, in this case, is made of words, metaphors, interpretations, and/or readings. During the first years of my specialist training, early clinical experiences at the bedside of severely anorexic patients who were often also psychotic enabled me to understand the nutritive value of words (rather than the calorie count of food) aimed at an adequate emotional diet required in the relationship with these young patients. I can safely say that I found this again in my work with schizophrenic patients: the therapeutic value of words as a means of recognition of and treatment for their mental suffering.

Another means of countertransference aimed at promoting a "nutritive" relationship with the patient concerns his or her need for protection. This countertransference is often expressed in the analyst's tendency to "protect" the psychotic individual from risks and dangers from the social environment as well as from his or her own behavior, behavior that is potentially damaging to himself or herself as well as to others (with the social and sometimes legal repercussions that arise from it). Behavior involving alcohol and other drug abuse sometimes associated (e.g., in conditions of socioeconomic deprivation) with risky sexual behavior (promiscuity, prostitution, unprotected sex) is common for those who experience psychosis at a young age. The patient may use these as a strategy—even though often harmful in the long term—for confronting the existential anguish and experience of psychotic fragmentation. These behaviors give health care professionals an image of the patient as a vulnerable individual both mentally and physically, inducing in the analyst not only hypercontrolling and symbiotic behaviors (i.e., deriving from unconscious collusion with historical dynamics already put in place by the patient's reference figures) but also healthy, protective measures aimed at establishing boundaries and behavioral limits, just as good-enough parents do when they try to establish rules in the interest of the health and psychophysical integrity of their child.

A less explicit variant of protective anaclitic countertransference emerges in the context of didactic supervision or in discussion groups about clinical cases (which mainly occur in residential homes or hospitals). In these situations, the analyst is seen almost to "defend" the behavior of one of his or her patients from the comments and direct interpretations of the supervisor or a colleague, just as parents would when faced with negative comments about, or more or less similar attacks on, their own child.

Similar dynamics can also be seen in clinical situations in which the therapist finds himself or herself justifying the psychotic individual's behavior deemed to be highly dysfunctional, if not frankly bizarre, by the patient's family. The therapist may try to offer them explanations and reassurance as well as to instill in them an understanding of the patient's problematic conduct.

Finally, that the individual in psychosis—contrary to what Freud (1963 [1917]) and, at least at first, Jaspers (1972) believed to be true—yearns for intimacy in his or her relationship with the therapist is demonstrated in the emergence in the therapist of countertransferential feelings of tacit love toward the patient. These may include the feeling of desiring the patient, anticipating or seeking a meeting, enjoying his or her presence, and feeling admiration for and pride in him or her.

The anaclitic nature of this type of countertransference is seen in the countertransferential position assumed by the analyst, which becomes that of a new parent, an older brother or sister, a relative, or a close friend who is able to deliberately feed and nourish the patient's need for relational intimacy. The patient is experienced, regardless of his or her chronological age, as a child, or in certain cases, as an adolescent on the threshold of adulthood (often actually the case in clinical practice with young adult patients). Unlike the historical experience of the individual with schizophrenia, anaclitic countertransference based on intimacy gives the therapist the opportunity to finally bring that trust, support, human contact, guidance, playfulness, and responsibility to the relationship, qualities that the patient in psychosis still needs in order to continue his or her psychodevelopmental journey toward individuation.

Clinical cases

Mr Blake

Mr Blake, in his fifties, had been well-known to local mental health services since the age of 17. He suffered from a severe form of paranoid schizophrenia with delusions of persecution and powerful auditory hallucinations that had led him to commit violent acts against others over the years.

From his medical records, it was clear that he had had numerous hospital admissions and had also spent, when he was around 30 years old, a long period on a high-security forensic psychiatric ward following a psychotic relapse with associated sexual disinhibition that culminated in an episode of attempted violence with a knife against his ex-girlfriend.

Mr Blake's history documented how he had not had any contact with his father from early childhood onward. When Mr Blake was a teenager, his Caribbean father moved abroad and died some years later. Mr Blake was raised only partly by his mother, who was also afflicted with chronic psychosis. He had spent most of his teenage years living with a foster family, and during that time his first behavioral problems emerged at school with verbal aggression and physical impulsivity aimed at one of his female teachers.

I met him for the first time in an outpatient clinic, a few days after his move from the ward to his home to continue psychiatric treatment with the home treatment team, with which I worked as a psychiatrist. In that first meeting, my consultation was limited to a quick evaluation of his mental state followed by taking a small blood sample to work out the dose of clozapine, an antipsychotic medication he had been taking for a number of years with periods of noncompliance and that helped him to control, although only partly, his hallucinatory experiences.

In a tiny phlebotomy room, I faced a black man with dreadlocks. He wore a pair of very dark sunglasses. He was roughly 6" 2' tall and weighed around 266 pounds. I asked him to take a seat, and, while I was preparing the collection tube for the sample, something worrying slowly filled the room. Paradoxically, it was not his enormous frame or the relatively tight space in which we found ourselves but his odd hilarity, almost constant sniggers that were either interrupted with long silences or with a stream of disconnected phrases spoken at a barely audible level.

I started to feel uncomfortable in the room. I had become suddenly slow, repetitive in my movements; I carried on nervously looking for gloves; I had got the needle but my fingers had suddenly started to tremble; I was visibly clumsy. Although I had my back to Mr Blake, I felt the weight of his gaze on me. I was frightened for a moment, without an objective reason for being so, that he might actually get closer or even attack me from behind. I could still hear the patient behind me whispering something, but to my ears these were now indistinct sounds and rumbling noises. I finally found the gloves, which were in fact right under my nose. I got rid of the needle and took a new one. I took hold of the tourniquet, turned jerkily, and assuming a calm demeanor I did not feel, I asked him:

(P = Patient, T = Therapist)

T: Do you have good veins?"

P: "Do you have good manners?"

T: "I'm sorry, what?"

P: "I good veins, yes and you good manners," he declared.

T: "Oh yes, of course," as a nervous laugh escaped me.

P: "Helios, Hermes, Aphrodite, Gaia, Ares, Zeus, Chronos, Uranus, Pluto … we are surrounded … 136472 MakeMake … Make Love Make Love … 136472 where is the love? Stop procreation … Pluto, Uranus, Chronos, Zeus, Ares, Gaia, Aphrodite, Hermes, Helios … 136472 MakeMake … Make Love Make Love …136472 Where is the love? Stop procreation …136472 … Where is the love? Stop procreation."

It took me a few minutes to understand that he was talking about the solar system. Mr Blake had substituted the names of the planets with the names of the corresponding Greek gods, and only many weeks after that first meeting did I realize that he was familiar with the order of the different planets from the sun. Not only that, but he explained to me how MakeMake was the name of a dwarf planet discovered a decade earlier with the designated number of 136472. He talked about the end of the world, that aliens existed he was in no doubt, that these messages sent by aliens concerned all humanity and therefore also me. He was visibly hallucinating, as if he were listening to something and replying to these messages with incongruous laughter and sometimes touching his genitals in a stereotyped way.

The scene had become almost surreal. While I tried to stammer, "Can I come closer to take the sample?" he, hardly paying any attention, carried on holding out his bare forearm, relaxed the entire time, and added, "Give me your magnitude, I need your magnitude …"

He continued to repeat that there were aliens, that there had been a big explosion. Then all of a sudden my mobile phone started to ring. "Ohhhh, this is the alarm, this is the alarm," he began to shout. He made to stand up but with a movement of my hand I indicated to him, although frightened myself, that he should stay calm. In the meantime, on the other end of the phone was reception, who were asking me if everything was OK because they had noticed that the patient had not yet come out of the room. "Yes," I replied nervously, "We are safe and sound."

Mr Blake had already settled himself back in the chair. He stared at me for a moment, and with an inquiring look asked, "Spanish or Italian?" "Who? Me?" I asked. "Yes Doc, your accent … Are you Spanish or Italian?" I don't know what obscure motive (it must have been unconscious) prompted me to reply seriously and in a completely level tone of voice, "Martian, Mr Blake, I am a Martian." And then I added, "They were calling from space. They are asking if Mr Blake intends to have this blasted sample taken, and if afterward he'd like a cappuccino at the Cuban place around the corner!"

The room filled with thunderous and irrepressible laughter. And only then did I begin to breathe a sigh of relief.

It was the beginning of a series of verbal transactions in which Mr Blake wanted to know which part of Italy I came from before moving on to a very articulate discussion of the Italian mafia, various more or less scientific hypotheses about the existence of aliens, and the gods of Mount Olympus, during which he demonstrated a vast knowledge of mythology.

Mr Blake's persecutory voices had generated over time an entire cosmogony taking the form of planets and Greek gods. It quickly became clear to me that this was primarily the journey that was awaiting me if I really wanted to get involved with Mr Blake's voices, his "mission on Earth," and therefore the cosmogonic system he had unconsciously contrived in order to survive his persecutory anguish and, paradoxically, to communicate it to other people.

As part of home treatment, I was able to see Mr Blake again at our office roughly three times a week for between 40 and 90 minutes each time over a period of almost four months. During our meetings, his personal account of his life and his own experience of psychosis revolved mainly around his relationship with his mother, whom he described as an extremely abusive person who was herself affected by a schizophrenic-like psychosis. His mother had often stopped him from attending school, regularly fearing, delusionally, that someone would harm her, particularly when she was alone in the house. "I had become her bodyguard," he told me once, quoting his mother's own phrase. Up to the age of 10, Mr Blake also suffered from enuresis and sometimes encopresis. He also remembered episodes from the past during which he was repeatedly beaten by his mother with a belt, and as time went on, he had reacted to this by becoming sexually aroused. He used to masturbate while thinking about the physical abuse carried out by his mother, which had, in part, led to a disorder in his sexual identity. Mr Blake also talked about a relationship with a girlfriend, stating that he had hit her because she was using him and sleeping with other men.

Mr Blake's personality, in accordance with the structural diagram of paranoid schizophrenia (Figure 3.3 in Chapter 3), reflected a premature and prolonged Parent exclusion deriving from: (1) an emotionally distant, physically unavailable, neglectful father; and (2) an emotionally and physically abusive, symbiotic mother. In addition, his mother's paranoid psychosis severely impacted her son's psychosocial development during childhood and adolescence, and he historically responded with affective indifference and emotional withdrawal, deviant sexual arousal, psychomotor agitation, and later violence as an ultimate strategy to contain his mother's confused Child.

Mr Blake's aggressive and sexually disinhibited behavior was later extended through persecutory-adversarial transference toward other female figures (teachers, girlfriends, mental health professionals).

It was the combination of the structural absence of the paternal Parent— what Lacan (1993 [1956], 2006 [1958]) would have called the "foreclosure of the name-of-the-father" or "lack of paternal metaphor"—in the presence of a symbiotically abusing mother that configured the particular paranoid structure of Mr Blake's personality.

Despite the Parent exclusion (P_2 and P_1) taking place to avoid retraumatizing the Child, the excluded maternal Parent in Mr Blake's case was still able to influence the patient's internal world through the process of contamination. This was evidenced by second- and third-person auditory hallucinations in the form of derogatory voices and persecutory delusions followed by aggressive and often sexually disinhibited behavior toward others, especially women.

Over the years, Mr Blake had developed a delusional system in which it was not his mother but "aliens" from interstellar space who were responsible for the interference in his thinking and even for his violent actions. To these "evil" aliens, of which he was deeply and unshakeably afraid, he had attributed multiple voices and "messages of death" that were sent to him almost every day. As a result, talking about planets, galaxies, the origins and the end of the world had become a way for him to allow a "terrestrial" interlocutor to approach his inner world, even though this might appear to other people to be light years away, chaotic, and alien in itself.

Following his last discharge from the home treatment team in Lambeth, I often encountered Mr Blake, whether in the waiting room in the outpatient department or on the streets around Brixton where he lived. Every time we bumped into each other, he greeted me with a "Hey Doc! Any messages from space for me?" When his question was also accompanied by a grin, I knew that he was in a good place, that an Adult part of him was able to keep an eye on his anguished Child. And on those occasions I always said to him, "Yes, of course, they asked me if you want a cappuccino from the Cuban guy round the corner." And in general that was my way of having a conversation with Mr Blake somewhere more informal while making sure we talked about his inner world and bringing him closer, a little at a time, to everyday reality.

Abena

Abena was around 19 when she was admitted to the acute psychiatry ward on the Lambeth Early Onset unit. I was in my second year of transactional analytic training, and I did not yet have a strong grasp of the theoretical and methodological ideas underpinning the psychodynamic treatment of psychotic patients.

Abena was first taken to a local accident and emergency (A&E) department by her employer after an initial episode of what appeared at first to be panic attacks. She had only been seen once before about three months previously as an outpatient in the local mental health department for an earlier problem concerning insomnia associated with weight loss. She had refused to take any medication and did not attend subsequent appointments. However, after a second, violent episode of acute anxiety in which Abena had appeared confused and overcome by anguish connected with the fear of having "something strange in my stomach," she was sent again to A&E and then admitted to the psychiatry department for a more thorough diagnosis and assessment for therapy treatment.

On meeting Abena for the first time on the ward, I was faced with a black woman, of medium height, with very short hair and an unkempt appearance who seemed younger than her actual chronological age. She wore very wide black trousers and a fairly outlandish, clearly dirty blouse covered in a harlequin pattern but with rather faded colors. She was visibly in anguish, trembling, at times perplexed. Her large lips were barely moving, almost shut tight, although one could still see her white teeth in a mask-like face that stared at the floor. Our meeting took place in her hospital room and lasted a couple of hours. What immediately captured my attention, and somehow kept my curiosity alive during the whole of that meeting, was Abena's posture: I found her on one side of the bed on the floor, so curled up she looked as if she was in the fetal position, with both feet flat on the floor, her knees bent up to her chest, and her long, thin arms wrapped round them.

The doctor who had admitted her and the ward nurses were concerned about her nutritional state and suspected that she had not been eating enough for days. She had not touched any food since her arrival in clinic, even though her tray of lunch was on the windowsill along with at least three 50cl bottles, still sealed: two of water and one of Coca Cola.

I looked at her emaciated form and wondered how we would best be able to help her over the coming days. I introduced myself and immediately voiced my concerns:

(T = Therapist)

T: "Hello Abena. My name is Zefiro, and I am an Italian doctor working in this department, although usually I look after patients directly in their homes." (Silence)

T: "I have been called in because I know that you have lived in Italy, and perhaps we can communicate better in Italian. Is it OK if we talk in Italian?" (Silence. Abena maintained her fixed stare downward, unblinking.)

T: "I want you to know that you are currently safe in a hospital. It is 4 o'clock in the afternoon. We are here because we want to help you. No one here means you any harm." (More silence)

T: "We just want to understand what's going on and whether you are willing to share with us what you are thinking and feeling." (Another long silence during which the patient remained still and mute.)

T: "I am concerned about you at the moment. You look very thin and dehydrated."

Two interminable hours followed during which I gave up bit by bit my fairly halting attempts to elicit any form of response from Abena to my direct questions.

However, something paradoxical was being brought powerfully to my attention in that meeting with that young patient. It was something incredibly alive, which from that point on would typify how I entered into a relationship with the psychotic perplexity and almost ineffable existential anguish of many of these patients. That something was my own body. I became unexpectedly hyperconscious of my own body. All my movements seemed to me to suggest something powerfully insane if not frankly dangerous for Abena. While not wanting it to happen, I perceived my body doing something to Abena, and at the same time, I felt as if the entirety of Abena's posture, silence, face, and body was having a direct, and also inexpressible, impact on me. It took several years of clinical practice and study for me to give a name to this relational occurrence which today, almost inadvertently, I recognize as projective identification and counteridentification and, better still, bodily transference and countertransference. What happened was a rising state of unease within me, a sensation of both intolerable physical and mental discomfort, an unrest of the soul that induced me finally to stand up completely and slip away brokenly from the room.

With the consent of my colleagues on the ward, my line manager allowed me to come to the ward on a daily basis to attempt to engage Abena in some form of spoken dialogue. The following day I found Abena in the same position in which I had left her. I knew, however, from the doctor on night duty that the patient had independently put herself to bed, assumed the same seated position on the bed, and stubbornly remained awake, maintaining the same position for most of the night. It was clear, therefore, that the following morning she had reassumed the curled-up position on the floor before I arrived. I interpreted her behavior as her (unconscious) desire to wait again for someone to arrive (perhaps myself).

Her breakfast was there on the windowsill, untouched. Resolutely, perhaps also a little piqued, but without saying a word, I picked up a bottle of water and sat on the floor in front of her. Once again a long silence heralded my entrance into that special bodily dimension of my being, which I later discovered in Berne's concept of protocol and tissue-level experience. And precisely because of this interbodily experience, it was clear to me that I was facing a defined boundary that Abena had drawn around herself, in particular confining her body within a restricted space in a sort of mass of flesh and blood. But in that space I now saw her fragile self encamped, fragmented into countless faded colored pieces, just like her multicolored blouse. This self, despite its fragility, sought within the boundaries of a rigid posture a container and a containment (i.e., an ego), a nonplace place to be as a unity, to achieve an internal regrouping that was palpable and visible from the outside, visible at least to eyes that wanted to see and thus understand.

I tried to offer her the bottle of water as if through the invisible boundary that ran around her body, and Abena let out a high-pitched and sudden cry that made my heart literally jump in my chest. Almost like a conditioned reflex, I dropped the bottle on the ground not far from her feet. She grabbed it roughly, unscrewed the lid with her teeth, and started to empty it violently, shaking the container all over the place, soaking everything around her, visibly irritated, finally flinging the half-empty container at me. I was beginning to intuit how her body spoke and slowly got up and then sat down again, this time with an apple in my hand from her breakfast; it was a whole one. Quietly, this time deliberately, I put the apple down again near her toes, a bit concerned that she was shortly going to fling it at me. And what happened carried on sparking my interest. Abena brusquely brought the apple to her mouth, biting into it, and spitting one piece at a time all around her, and then getting rid of the core in the same way as she had got rid of the bottle: by hurling it directly at me.

Abena was no longer as perplexed as I initially thought. She was no longer mute but simply spoke a different language, that of her body. She herself was her body. Her mental pain had become body, cries, water, spitting, apple, chunks. Her ego was reduced to tiny drops of water, to pieces and chunks in the presence of an anonymous other, in the presence of the entire world, even though this was a world enclosed in a hospital room.

Without thinking, I instinctively collected up the water, gathering together the chunks of apple piece by piece. And I did it patiently and in the unexpected hope of repairing something that seemed broken into many bits, spread in different directions. In doing this, I used my hands and bent down a number of times. It was my improvised rite of reparation and hope. Abena stayed still, seemingly paying no attention to anything.

I sat then in silence, huddled in front of her for almost another hour with the remains of her world in pieces in front of me. I then thought to get her simply milk and hot coffee for lunch, this time in a bowl, and also apple puree in a bowl that the nurses placed by her feet. Thus, with the bowls held in her own hands, Abena began to feed herself again, eating fruit and vegetable purees, soups, broths, and also water, a little at a time—as if the bowl had something of the reparatory about it, welcoming and perhaps even mystical and unifying.

A social worker from the borough of Lambeth where Abena had earlier lived, and who had been involved with Abena in her early adolescence, was able to get hold of important details from her history, which was much more traumatic than I had been led to believe at first. Abena originally came from Ghana and had first landed in Italy, specifically in Sicily, about 15 years earlier on a migrant boat from Libya. She had been taken into the care of the social services and finally adopted by a rich family in the Sicilian hinterland. She was given the opportunity to learn Italian and complete, although with difficulty, her mandatory schooling.

Abena's own account of her personal history was initially rather sparse owing to her continued mutism as well as fairly frequent episodes during which she seemed clearly confused and absorbed in her internal world. These symptoms gradually improved after a number of weeks of treatment with a low dose of antipsychotic medication and mild therapy for insomnia.

Although she was reluctant to speak about her personal history, in the end she revealed that she had no memory of her biological parents, who had, according to her adoptive parents, "abandoned her in the sea" at about age four. She spoke in small fragments, session after session, about how her adoptive parents had separated when she was around 13 years old, and for roughly four years after that she went to live with the parents of her adoptive mother. The separation of her adoptive parents was accompanied by a fair amount of conflict and ended up with her father moving to the north of Italy while her mother had begun a relationship with a work colleague near Palermo. Over time, Abena and her adoptive parents lost contact with each other. During that period, intrusive and bizarre thoughts began to surface, such as believing she was responsible for the "disappearance" of her adoptive parents, and the idea that the parents of her adoptive mother were "complicit" in this "kidnap," as she herself called it. During our sessions she continued to maintain that she was certain that her parents' disappearance was due to her. As time went on, impostors had sought her out by telephone, and subsequently even by email, claiming to be her "real" adoptive parents. She says she did not shy away from meeting, if only rarely, these "supposed parents" and did so usually at the house of her adoptive grandparents. She does not remember, however, what they talked about on those occasions. What was certain is that she kept to herself the "secret of the kidnapping" for several years, "pretending to be normal" until she moved to London with the aim of finding work and learning English. Until a week before her admission to the ward, she was working as a cashier at a chain of Italian pizzerias in London.

I was unable to find out more about what happened to Abena in recent months apart from the circumstances of the acute disorder that had prompted her employer to take her to A&E.

When I reminded her that in the A&E at St. Thomas's Hospital she had stated to the doctors that she had "something strange in her stomach," she suddenly seemed to remember an episode, some days before her admission, in which she had heard her own stomach "talking."

(P = Patient, T = Therapist)

T: "I'm not sure I've understood that correctly. You mean you heard your stomach gurgling?"
P: "No, no. My stomach is talking to me!"
T: "Talking to you?"
P: "Yes, my stomach speaks, and only I can hear it."
T: "And what does it tell you?"

Long silence.

T: "Does the voice in your stomach remind you of someone you know?"

P: "No. They are nobody's voices."

T: "There is more than one voice? More than one voice that you don't recognize?"

P: "Yes, it is a stomach of a thousand voices," she laughs incongruously.

T: "And you don't know what they are saying to you?"

P: "No. That is … "

T: "That is, they don't tell you anything or they tell you not to say?"

P: "They say that I mustn't speak," she said turning her eyes toward a corner of the room.

T: "Do you think staying silent has something to do with not revealing your secret?"

Silence.

Abena's psychosis, in line with the structural diagram of schizoid psychoses, had its own historical (and therefore structural) roots in the fundamental and very early absence of a good-enough parental role, culminating in original exclusions of the Parent (P_0, P_1), and was able to translate electively into preverbal and bodily manifest actions of her experience of her self. In fact, the phenomenology of her acute psychosis was a clear expression of a dissociative Child and consisted of a somatic and auditory hallucination about her "talking stomach" because her mouth was supposed to stay shut and presumably keep the inexpressible secret about the absence of the Parent. At the same time, however, her Child was paradoxically searching for a new interlocutor, for affective and physical containment via a somatic transference and yearning-for-the-Parent transactions. It is worth noting that during her stay in the hospital, other members of staff often experienced strong feelings of countertransference in wanting to care for her because she appeared like a small, terrified child seeking a lot of reassurance, affection, and protection.

During her clinical conversations with me in the hospital, which were followed by regular sessions initially with the home treatment team and then in the outpatient clinic around three times per week for a period of about a year, Abena started to recognize, if only partially, the somatic hallucinations to be a direct expression of her internal object world and her own past traumatic relational experiences. Her Child had preferred to create a bodily narrative of the latter in which the experience of her "talking stomach" indicated in a single verbal expression the embodied sense of her mental suffering.

References

Anderson, F. S. (2008). *Bodies in treatment: The unspoken dimension*. New York, NY: The Analytic Press.

Anzieu, D. (1989). *The skin ego: A psychoanalytic approach to the self.* New Haven, CT: Yale University Press.

Berne, E. (1970). *Sex in human loving.* New York, NY: Penguin Books.

Berne, E. (1975a). *The structure and dynamics of organizations and groups.* New York, NY: Grove Press. (Original work published 1963)

Berne, E. (1975b). *Transactional analysis in psychotherapy: A systematic individual and social psychiatry.* London: Souvenir Press. (Original work published 1961)

Berne, E. (1975c). *What do you say after you say hello? The psychology of human destiny.* London: Corgi. (Original work published 1972)

Berne, E. (1977). Primal images and primal judgment. In E. Berne, P. McCormick (Ed.), *Intuition and ego states: The origins of transactional analysis* (pp. 67–97). San Francisco, CA: TA Press. (Original work published 1955)

Bick, E. (1968). The experience of the skin in early object relations. *International Journal of Psychoanalysis*, 29, 484–486.

Bick, E. (2002). Further considerations on the function of the skin in early object relations. In A. Briggs (Ed.), *Surviving space: Papers on infant observation* (pp. 60–71). London: Karnac Books. (Original work published 1986)

Bion, W. R. (1977). *Learning from experience.* London: William Heinemar. (Original work published 1962)

Bion, W. R. (1984). *Second thoughts: Selected papers on psychoanalysis.* London: Karnac Books. (Original work published 1967)

Bleuler, E. (1950). *Dementia praecox or the group of schizophrenias* (Monograph Series on Schizophrenia 1) (J. Zinkin, Trans.). New York, NY: International Universities Press. (Original work published 1911)

Bloom, K. (2006). *The embodied self: Movement and psychoanalysis.* London: Karnac Books.

Bollas, C. (1987). *The shadow of the object: Psychoanalysis of the unthought known.* New York, NY: Columbia University Press.

Bollas, C. (2013). *Catch them before they fall: The psychoanalysis of breakdown.* London: Routledge.

Bucci, W. (1997a). *Psychoanalysis and cognitive science: A multiple code theory.* New York, NY: Guilford Press.

Bucci, W. (1997b). Symptoms and symbols: A multiple code theory of somatization. *Psychoanalytic Inquiry*, 17, 151–172.

Bucci, W. (2008). The role of bodily experience in emotional organization: New perspectives on the multiple code theory. In F. S. Anderson (Ed.), *Bodies in treatment: The unspoken dimension* (pp. 51–76). New York, NY: The Analytic Press.

Burns, T., Knapp, M., Catty, J., Healey, A., Henderson, J., Watt, H., & Wright, C. (2001). Home treatment for mental health problems: A systematic review. *Health Technology Assessment*, 5, 1–139.

Ciompi, L. (1982). *Affektlogik: Über die struktur der psyche und ihre entwicklung. Ein beitrag zur schizophrenieforschung.* Stuttgart: Klett-Cotta. [English version: *The psyche and schizophrenia: The bond between affect and logic* (D.L. Schneider, Trans.). Cambridge, MA, London: Harvard University Press, 1988]

Ciompi, L. (2003). Reflections on the role of emotions in consciousness and subjectivity, from the perspective of affect logic. *Consciousness and Emotion*, 4, 181–196.

Clarkson, P. (1992). *Transactional analysis psychotherapy: An integrated approach.* London: Routledge.

Cornell, W. F. (2008a). "My body is unhappy": Somatic foundations of script and script protocol. In W. F. Cornell, *Explorations in transactional analysis: The Meech Lake papers* (pp. 159–170). Pleasanton, CA: TA Press.

Cornell, W. F. (2008b). Self in action: The bodily basis of self-organization. In F. S. Anderson (Ed.), *Bodies in treatment: The unspoken dimension* (pp. 29–50). New York, NY: The Analytic Press.

Cornell, W. F. (2015). *Somatic experience in psychoanalysis and psychotherapy: In the expressive language of the living.* London: Routledge.

Cornell, W. F., & Hargaden, H. (2005). *From transactions to relations: The emergence of a relational tradition in transactional analysis.* Chadlington: Haddon Press.

Cornell, W. F., & Landaiche, N. M., III (2006). Impasse and intimacy: Applying Berne's concept of script protocol. *Transactional Analysis Journal, 36,* 196–213.

Cornell, W. F., & Landaiche, N. M., III (2008). Nonconscious processes and self-development: Key concepts from Eric Berne and Christopher Bollas. *Transactional Analysis Journal, 38,* 200–218.

Damasio, A. (1996). *Descartes' error: Emotion, reason and the human brain.* New York, NY: Harper Collins. (Original work published 1994)

Damasio, A. (1999). *The feeling of what happens: Body and emotions in the making of consciousness.* New York, NY: Harcourt Brace.

English, F. (1988). Whither scripts? *Transactional Analysis Journal, 18,* 294–303.

Erskine, R. G. (2010). Life scripts: Unconscious relational patterns and psychotherapeutic involvement. In R. G. Erskine (Ed.), *Life scripts: A transactional analysis of unconscious relational patterns* (pp. 1–28). London: Karnac Books.

Federn, P. (1953). *Ego psychology and the psychoses.* London: Imago Publishing. (Original work published 1952)

Fernald, A. (1984). The perceptual and affective salience of mothers' speech to infants. In L. Feagans, C. Garvey, & R. Golinkoff (Eds.), *The origins and growth of communication* (pp. 5–29). Norwood, NJ: Ablex.

Fonagy, P., Gergely, G., Jurist, E. L., & Target, M. (2002). *Affect regulation, mentalization and the development of the self.* New York, NY: Other Press.

Fowlie, H., & Sills, C. (2011). *Relational transactional analysis: Principles in practice.* London: Karnac Books.

Freud, S. (1958). Three essays on the theory of sexuality. In J. Strachey (Ed. & Trans.), *The standard edition of the complete psychological works of Sigmund Freud* (Vol. 7, pp. 123–245). London: Hogarth Press. (Original work published 1905)

Freud, S. (1963). Lecture XXVII: Transference. In J. Strachey (Ed. & Trans.), *The standard edition of the complete psychological works of Sigmund Freud* (Vol. 16, pp. 431–447). London: Hogarth Press. (Original work published 1917)

Grinberg, L. (1979). Countertransference and projective counteridentification. *Contemporary Psychoanalysis, 15,* 226–247.

Grotstein, J. S. (1981). *Splitting and projective identification.* New York, NY: Jason Aronson.

Grotstein, J. S. (2005). Projective transidentification: An extension of the concept of projective identification. *International Journal of Psychoanalysis, 86,* 1051–1069.

Hargaden, H., & Sills, C. (2002). *Transactional analysis: A relational perspective.* Hove: Brunner-Routledge.

Heath, D. S. (2004). *Home treatment for acute mental disorders: An alternative to hospitalization.* New York, NY: Routledge.

Howell, E. F. (2002). Back to the states: Victim and abuser states in borderline personality disorder. *Psychoanalytic Dialogues*, 12, 921–957.

Howell, E. F., & Blizard, R. A. (2009). Chronic relational trauma disorder: A new diagnostic scheme for borderline personality and the spectrum of dissociative disorders. In P. F. Dell & J. A. O'Neil (Eds.), *Dissociation and the dissociative disorders: DSM-V and beyond* (pp. 495–510). New York, NY: Routledge.

Jaspers, K. (1972). *General psychopathology*. Manchester: Manchester University Press.

Johnson, S., Needle, J., Bindman, J., & Thornicocroft, G. (2008). *Crisis resolution and home treatment teams in mental health*. Cambridge: Cambridge University Press.

Klein, M. (1997). Envy and gratitude. In M. Klein, *Envy and gratitude and other works, 1946–1963* (pp. 176–235). London: Vintage. (Original work published 1957)

La Barre, F. (2001). *On moving and being moved: Nonverbal behavior in clinical practice*. Hillsdale, NJ: The Analytic Press.

Lacan, J. (1993). *The seminar of Jacques Lacan: The psychoses, 1955–1956* (Book 3) (J. A. Miller, Ed., & R. Grigg, Trans.). New York, NY: Norton. (Original work published 1956)

Lacan, J. (1998). *On feminine sexuality: The limits of love and knowledge, 1972–1973* (Book 20). (J. A. Miller, Ed., & B. Fink, Trans.). New York, NY: Norton. (Original work published 1972)

Lacan, J. (2006). On a question prior to any possible treatment of psychosis. In J. Lacan, J. A. Miller (Ed.), *Écrits: The first complete edition in English* (B. Fink, Trans.) (pp. 445–488). New York, NY: Norton. (Original work published 1958)

Laing, R. D. (1959). *The divided self: An existential study in sanity and madness*. London: Penguin Books.

Lemma, A. (2015). *Minding the body: The body in psychoanalysis and beyond*. London: Routledge.

Mancia, M. (2007). *Feeling the words: Neuropsychoanalytic understanding of memory and the unconscious*. London: Routledge.

Mellacqua, Z. (2014). Beyond symbiosis: The role of primal exclusion in schizophrenic psychosis. *Transactional Analysis Journal*, 44, 8–30.

Meltzer, D. (1975). Adhesive identification. *Contemporary Psychoanalysis*, 11, 289–310.

Moiso, C. (1985). Ego states and transference. *Transactional Analysis Journal*, 15, 194–201.

Nijenhuis, E. R. S. (1999). *Somatoform dissociation: Phenomena, measurement and theoretical issues*. Assen: Van Gorcum.

Ogden, T. (1992). *Projective identification and psychotherapeutic technique*. London: Karnac Books. (Original work published 1982)

Panksepp, J. (1998). *Affective neuroscience: The foundations of human and animal emotions*. New York, NY: Oxford University Press.

Panksepp, J. (2009). Brain emotional systems and qualities of emotional life: From animal models of affect to implications for psychotherapeutics. In D. Fosha, D. J. Siegel, & M. F. Solomon (Eds.), *The healing power of emotions: Affective neuroscience, development, and clinical practice* (pp. 1–26). New York, NY: Norton.

Perls, F. S., Hefferline, R. F., & Goodman, P. (1951). *Gestalt therapy: Excitement and growth in the human personality*. New York, NY: Julian Press.

Perry, B. D. (1999). The memory of states: How the brain stores and retrieves traumatic experience. In J. Goodwin & R. Attias (Eds.), *Splintered reflections: Images of the body in treatment* (pp. 9–38). New York, NY: Basic Books.

Racker, H. (1957). The meanings and uses of countertransference. *Psychoanalytic Quarterly*, 26, 303–357.

Resnik, S. (2005). *Glacial times: A journey through the world of madness.* New York, NY: Routledge.

Samuels, A. (2016). "I rebel, therefore we are" (Albert Camus): New political thinking on individual responsibility for group, society, culture, and planet. *Transactional Analysis Journal*, 46, 101–108.

Schore, A. N. (2001). Neurobiology, developmental psychology and psychoanalysis: Convergent findings on the subject of projective identification. In J. Edwards (Ed.), *Being alive: Building on the work Anne Alvarez* (pp. 57–74). London: Brunner-Routledge.

Schore, A. N. (2003). *Affect regulation and repair of the self.* New York, NY: Norton.

Schore, A. N. (2012). *The science of the art of psychotherapy.* New York, NY: Norton.

Spotnitz, H. (1985). *Modern psychoanalysis of the schizophrenic patient: Theory of the technique* (2nd edn). New York, NY: Human Sciences Press.

Stuthridge, J. (2006). Inside out: A transactional analysis model of trauma. *Transactional Analysis Journal*, 36, 270–283.

Tustin, F. (1990). *The protective shell in children and adults.* London: Karnac Books.

Wheeler, C., Lloyd-Evans, B., Churchard, A., Fitzgerald, C.Fullarton, K., Mosse, L., & Johnson, S. (2015). Implementation of the crisis resolution team model in adult mental health settings: A systematic review. *BioMed Central Psychiatry*, 15, 74.

Winnicott, D. W. (1975). Hate in the countertransference. In D. W. Winnicott, *Through paediatrics to psychoanalysis: Collected papers* (pp. 194–203). New York, NY: Basic Books.

Woollams, S., & Brown, M. (1978). *Transactional analysis.* Dexter, MI: Huron Valley Institute.

5

THE NAKED SELF

In healthy development, somewhat paradoxically, the Other is the crucible within which, and in relation to which, the self of the individual is shaped. The Other, indeed, inhabits both the internal and the external world, nature, the cosmos, and reality in general. The self exists through the Other and for the Other. So, what is the Other? And, as a consequence, what is the self? And why the two are so intimately connected?

The Other is primarily any other human being but also any other living creature, even a physical object or a place, an element of nature that happens to be unconsciously infused by the developing individual with a special long-lasting significance. This special, often enduring, connectedness is what allows the self to either grow or perish. This is why the Other ultimately coincides, on the one hand, with the unconscious internalization—through introjection and identification—within the developing ego of multiple idiosyncratic relation-ships between the self and any significant Other(s), and, on the other hand, with the projection—essentially through transference—outside one's ego onto new others (be they persons, physical objects, places, etc.) of the *vestigia* (i.e., historical traces) of such internal (i.e., intrapsychic) multiplicity. The Other serves a potentially regulatory or dysregulatory function for the ego according to the nature of the multiple relationships the Other has with the self throughout development.

In transactional analysis terms, we can conclude that structurally the "real self" primarily originates and resides in the Child. The Child ego state is, in fact, the part of our personality that is felt by us as "me-through-the-Other" from the beginning of our intrauterine life onward (see Chapter 1). As such, the self is a much freer entity than the ego, being able to move within and through the ego. However, one's experience of having a coherent sense of self depends on the development and quality of one's ego boundaries (Federn, 1953 [1952]).

This way of thinking suggests that there is a clear difference between the nature of the self and the ego. The self corresponds to the multifaceted experience of the ego in continuous exchange with internal and external reality, including, above all, the psychological reality of other people, but also of animals, concrete objects, places, nature, and the universe in general (Bollas, 2002 [1995], 2006 [1992]). Consequently, the self, as the "real" representative of the (inter)subjective psyche, is a diffuse and much larger entity than the ego. In contrast, the ego is a condensed plurality of states that are inherently coherent (i.e., ego states). The ego is, therefore, a complex plurality of body-mind states that consists of multiple conscious, preconscious, unconscious, and nonconscious systems. The main aim of the ego is to use its boundaries to provide coherence and organization for self-experience. In transactional analysis terms, if the Adult ego state identifies phenomenologically with the "I" (pronoun) of spoken and internal dialogue—that is to say, "the representative of the ego in consciousness" (Bollas, 2015, p. 189)—then the Child ego state is the "real self" or my-self. That is, it is the "signature" of one's being and, more precisely, the representative of the ego in relation to the historical Other and to external reality from the beginning of experiential life.

In summary, the evolutionary task of the Adult is integration, whereas the fundamental objective of the Child is self-integrity and therefore individuation.

Berne (1975a [1961]) clearly and meaningfully placed psychotic pathology exactly "on the boundary" between the Adult and the Child, between the "me" and the "self." He thereby inferred the derivation of the symptomatic manifestations of psychosis from a pathology of the Adult-Child boundary and therefore the ego-self boundary:

> Lesions of the boundary between the Adult and the Child may give rise to any of a special group of symptoms which may be called "boundary symptoms": feelings of unreality, estrangement, depersonalization, jamais vu, déja vu, and their analogues, such as the well-known déja raconté. ... If the Child is the "real Self," they become part of the psychotic array.
>
> (pp. 63–64)

In contrast to Berne's hypothesis, I propose that the structural determinant of schizophrenic psychosis is in pathology of the boundaries within the Child ego state—here designated as the *proper self*. It is the thickening of the external boundary of the Child-self (the excluding Child or C_2) that determines the exclusion of an Adult that has been traumatized and/or is not yet sufficiently developed (nonintegrated A_2). This makes it, in turn, responsible for the rather extensive impairment in reality testing and finally contributes to the alienation of the self from the external world.

At the same time, the increasing rigidity, through exclusion, of the external boundary of the Child ego state makes it particularly susceptible to "sclerosis of the boundary" (Berne, 1975a [1961], p. 66) until it splits in several parts or fragments. Such splits are made possible, among other reasons, due to the fracturing of internal boundaries of the Child-self (described in previous chapters in terms of vertical and horizontal splitting and the fragmented Child). It is possible, then, to view schizophrenic phenomenology—with its delusions, hallucinations, loss of a feeling of reality, hypochondriacal collapse, adherence to the Other, intrusiveness from the Other, and so on—from a structural perspective linked, in this case, also to sclerosis and multiple splitting of the Child ego state internal boundaries.

The resulting fragmentation brings to the surface what lies in the depths of the psychotic individual's psyche, which has not yet reached full adult development (classically represented in transactional analysis as the tripartite or pluripartite personality). I call this deep layer of being *the naked self* and offer the following clinical examples to illustrate its nature and functions in mental health and, specifically, schizophrenic pathology.

Jane

When the nurses called me to carry out an emergency assessment of Jane at her house, I found a young woman in her second episode of schizophrenic psychosis, huddled on the floor of her bedroom, completely naked, distressed, screaming, trembling, and drenched in her own urine. Jane was in a corner of the room, her expression was terrified. Her head seemed to be almost squashed between her narrow shoulders, which formed a trembling "V" shape. Her cries, the indistinct sounds of mental pain, had become rhythmic, as if she were trying to make herself and us aware of the desperate cry in her being.

It was not possible to engage Jane in conversation. Two other nurses had arrived and watched the unfolding scene, waiting for me to say something or to prescribe a sedative before transferring her to the hospital. I remained silent in front of Jane, overwhelmed, uncertain. A small part of me remained, nonetheless, listening. I made up my mind to remove the sheet from the bed, approached her, and wrapped the sheet around her shoulders and down around her waist. I ended up almost tentatively hugging her, holding her between my arms until she stopped trembling. Nurse Charlotte gently led the patient to the bathroom to deal with her personal needs. I could hear the nurse's voice reassuring Jane with simple words: "Come here, come here, it's nothing to worry about," "It's OK, I'm with you," "Let's get you into a nice warm bath," "No one is going to hurt you." Jane allowed herself to be reassured gently without the need for any forced treatment. She passively accepted being taken to Lambeth Hospital for a period of inpatient stay that lasted about two months.

I did not see Jane again after that, but the scene in her house left an indelible impression on me. Going back to those few minutes together, which my own psyche registered as an incredibly long time, I asked myself what, or who, or which part of Jane's being confronted me. I asked myself if what I saw, to borrow from Winnicott (1965), was Jane's "false self," and if so, what had happened to her presumed "true self"—or, vice versa, if what I had seen had been the truest part of her being, her "true self" or her Natural Child, to use Berne's expression? If so, then I hoped that a false self or a more or less Adapted Child of hers would appear on the scene by putting an end to that unbearable anguish.

What I actually experienced is what one cannot help but feel when faced with a frightened, crying little child needing the Other. When applied to Jane, Winnicott's distinction between true self and false self—and likewise Berne's differentiation between Natural Child and Adapted Child—was not enough. I therefore arrived at the hypothesis that distinguishing between the true self and the false self during active schizophrenic psychoses is not the issue. What the analyst is confronted with during psychotic processes is, in fact, a pre-egoic dimension of existence in which the psychotic individual con-*fuses* the self with the other-than-self, waiting for the ego to (re)establish itself first of all to falsify reality. And to falsify reality means to falsify first the Other's reality until a vision of the Other develops as other-than-self. In fact, the concept of a Natural or Free Child ego state, like that of a true self, implies that there is somewhere an essence of being human that can be considered to be separate from the nuclear relationship with the Other—understood as past Other, present Other, and future Other.

Instead, in line with the psychodevelopmental perspective discussed here, I suggest that the human psyche be considered nonunitary in origin, consisting rather of a chaotic multiplicity of body-mind states initially lacking an internal organization (i.e., C_0 and C_1). It is only by means of progressively internalized regulatory Others (i.e., P_0 and P_1) that, in healthy development, this initial inner discontinuity of being organizes itself into a more coherent structure. I call the earliest version of this ego structure a *pretending ego*. It is an infantile Adult ego or an Adult within the Child (i.e., A_0 and A_1) that acts toward, transacts with, and attracts the idiosyncratic attention of reference others as if it were a "little adult" among "proper" grown-ups.

In healthy conditions, the developing child would finally discover that he or she exists as a separate experiencing being while becoming aware, at the same time, that he or she is also an object in the world. This is a painful, but also playful, discovery in which the evolving ego assumes a more relational stance based on a preconscious, and then a more conscious, I-You distinction. From these inter-egoic relationships between the child and his or her reference others, the first psychological games and even script decisions originate. As such, this pretending ego is both a mental structure and a relational experience. As a mental structure, it accounts for the experience of continuity and coherence of one's emerging sense of self; as a relational dimension, it is both a source and a recipient of healthy narcissistic feelings, such as those provided by relationships with sensitive and responsive caregivers.

In contrast, schizophrenic pathology, perhaps more than any other, demonstrates how the person's sense of an unintegrated self, especially as experienced in the midst of a psychotic breakdown, strongly relates to the lack of the healthy narcissistic investment of a pretending ego. Again, in my view, this may reflect a defective internalization and/or imply a distorted representation of the Other(s) mainly for defensive and, therefore, adaptive purposes. This psychodynamic process has been described previously in terms of the Parent's exclusion(s) (see Chapter 3). With no real birth of the Other as other-than-self, the child's ego fails to develop as a pluripartite (P_1-A_1-C_1) ego. This failure is, however, not fatal because it puts the subject in search of the Other and, therefore, of himself or herself.

The encounter with Jane brought me to a new experiential awareness, that of her somehow unconsciously creating a sort of "environment baby," that is, as an infantile dimension of her-and-me being in a reciprocal relationship. Her naked self was somehow asking for a more profound recognition, a more radical permission to exist and to belong to life and to others at large.

This naked self exists separately from the establishment of a Natural Child and/or Adapted Child, thereby avoiding a division into a true self/false self that, among other things, is moralistic (or Parent-like). The naked self is a psychological reality that persists throughout life. It mumbles, fumbles, stumbles, and when put under threat, easily trembles and even crumbles. At the same time, it is continuously searching for an idiom of its own, for an intentional gesture or a step forward yet to be made, for a place where it can rest and live less precariously. In acting this way, the naked self resists the moral law of the internal Parent and stumbles precipitously out of external reality with the result that its Adult becomes easily lost or never sufficiently ready (A_0 and A_1). It begs the Other for permission to exist and digest its existential suffering, its fear of living like its fear of psychological death, of breaking down.

The naked self is, above all, a body-self (C_0) searching for its own ego. It encapsulates the vitality of the Child, sharing with the Other a vital base for existence or "a deeply engaged relationship which contains room for conflict, aggression, phantasy, insecurity, and uncertainty in addition to security and empathic attunement" (Cornell, 2015, p. 117).

From the start of intrauterine life, the naked self depends on the mother's body—seen as the big, original Other—and on her body-ego (maternal protocol) as well as the body-ego of significant others (parental protocol of the father and caregivers) for its future survival and its own "birth" as the Somatic Child (C_1). It passes through the first phases of neonatal life and the beginning of infancy to go on and develop fully throughout life. The naked self's destiny is to transcend, by means of primitive senses, the boundaries of its own body and those of the Other and to come, irrevocably, into contact with its own internal reality and external reality, with the finite and the infinite simultaneously. As such, the naked self is as open to death as to life, to illness as to health, to madness as to creativity, to fragmentation as to integrity, to collapse as to (re)birth, to con-fusion as to intimacy. The naked self thus embodies all the potentialities of being in its biological, psychological, relational, and even spiritual expressions according to the phases of ego development throughout the whole course of an individual's life.

The discussion that follows concerns the fate of the naked self in psychotic processes and which ways are open and which instead need to be opened in order to find such a naked self during therapy with individuals affected by schizophrenia.

Time and subjectivity

During states of psychotic breakdown with significant and evident disruption of self-experience—clinically visible as ego fragmentation in the areas of the individual's intellectual, bodily-emotional, behavioral and social-relational functioning—there is often a gap, a discontinuity, something unexpected hidden behind an "I don't know" or a "Nothing" comment from the patient. It may be a small thing that has caused a sudden, and at times even sinister, disturbance in the person's apparently normal, everyday stream of life, dramatically altering its course.

On the other hand, in cases of psychosis in which the onset is more gradual, recognizing the warning signs can take time because of the insidious appearance, for example, of a subtle thought disorder and rather bizarre changes in behavior, hesitations in speech, an unusual slowness and/or clumsiness of movement, and a growing feeling of estrangement from one's own self and external reality. Eventually, the person may enter some sort of pre-dissociative and dissociative states that are not always recognizable to the patient's family, friends, or acquaintances. In these cases, reconstructing the events that led up to the crisis, or even investigating the patient's psychobiography, must be postponed or sought, when possible, from the family and caregivers, at least those who might be able to provide extra information about the past and recent circumstances of the individual's life.

Whether faced with active psychosis or paucisymptomatic forms of schizophrenia, the main task of the transactional analyst is to guide the patient in crisis through a process of active grounding in reality. The analytic setting must, therefore, be conducive to careful inquiry into and emotional participation with the significant events in the patient's life, with attention paid to any details that may have disrupted the fluid continuity of the individual's existence, his or her "real self," to use Berne's meaningful term. During this exploratory phase, the analyst should try to restore a sense of agency to these patients when exploring their history, affirming the subjective credibility of their mental (including dreams), relational, physical, and even spiritual (when made explicit) experiences as well as their fragile relationship with reality.

When working with a patient in active psychosis, the grounding in reality involves another way of using spatiotemporal orientation, which in this case takes the form of a proper ordering—actually in space and time—of the person's recent life events. Painstakingly researching information about the presumed "nonevent event" that preceded the crisis allows the therapist to coconstruct as well as analyze meanings connected with the circumstances of the person's actual life, circumstances that become intertwined with pre-conscious and unconscious traumatic memories from infancy and pre-adolescence. It is during infancy, and even back as far as intrauterine psychobiological development, that preverbal and protomental experiences in the knowledge of self, others, and life in general are said to occur, that "unthought known" that Bollas (1987) wrote about and that in transactional analysis Berne initially defined as "primal protocol" (Berne, 1975a [1961], 1975b [1972], 1977 [1966]).

Often, even in more contemporary clinical settings, the opportunity for patients to access their traumatic protocol experiences is taken away by rapid hospitalization and aggressive use of antipsychotic medications. This practice too often results in patients' meanings remaining mostly inacces-sible, or even being eventually lost, behind their first psychotic crisis. This can lead many of them to suffer a progressive loss of a coherent narrative of their own unusual experiences (including hallucinations) while such experi-ences create a violent barrage of thoughts. Patients' progressive lack of coherence in thinking, and at times also of action, is often an indication of their subsequent *de-lirare* (from the Latin *delirāre*, made up of "dē-" and a derivative of līra *"furrow"*), that is, "going off the furrow" of the logical-rational associations of their own ideas.

Whether this manifests as patients' selective mutism in the face of incessant questions from their interlocutor, or whether they go into an unstoppable logorrhea (at times culminating in a "word salad"), the result is a desperate attempt to cope with an ineffable existential anguish brought about by the idea "I no longer know who I am." They evacuate their very self somewhere else: now in their own body, now in the Other, now in the body of the Other. These indescribable experiences of the patient's internal suffering, which are initially expressed physically—for example, in the form of polysensory (i.e., visual, tactile, and even olfactory) hallucinations—soon acquire features of a panic situation. This tends to affect the movements of the patient's body as well, movements that are experienced as happening outside the patient's own volition, as if they were directed or even remotely controlled by external forces or entities (including the therapist). By the same processes of psychotic influence that stem from a pathology of ego boundaries and their increasing fragility, thoughts are also placed elsewhere (thought withdrawal, thought broadcasting) or seem to come from outside their own head (thought inser-tion and telepathy) or become otherwise alien colonizers of their own mind. I call these "nobody's thoughts," playing with the idea of "no-body thoughts"—that is, disembodied thoughts or thoughts that run the risk of becoming dissociated from bodily-emotional life but that are full of primary existential meanings harkening back to the first phases of the individual's life.

It is precisely at this point in the analysis that the therapist can (or not) make a therapeutic choice that will affect the direction of the analysis itself and thereby the quality of the patient's future life. Rather than simply empathizing with the individual's psychotic experiences, the therapist can courageously choose to undertake, together with the patient, a risky reediting of protocol aspects of the individual's psychobiography with the aim of coconstructing new meanings to deal with the apparent incomprehensibility of the person's current crisis. A therapeutic choice of this kind is a function of the analyst's intuition, originally propounded by Berne, as well as being strongly in line with his deconfusion methodology predominantly aimed at the cure (understood as care and cure together) of the patient's Child ego state.

In work with psychotic subjects, grounding in reality—that is, the reality of the patient's actually lived events—takes time and often requires significant changes to the more usual aspects of therapy, such as rather fixed time boundaries (i.e., about 50–60 minutes) and a more or less variable frequency of sessions per week (also depending on various therapeutic approaches, not only those common in transactional analysis). The quality of this grounding process also depends on the level of commitment shown by the therapist and on the type of organizational context in which the work is done (hospital, outpatient clinic, private practice, part of a multidisciplinary home treatment team, etc.). In the end, the ultimate aim is to better facilitate the analytic process by creating the best conditions for a mutual (analyst's and patient's) understanding of the patient's predicament and instilling trust in patients that their own almost ineffable subjective experience can still be understood by means of their personal history and by focusing on the present time—both analytic and extra-analytic—of their lives.

Situating time in space

One of the main therapeutic techniques for bringing psychotic patients back to reality is to give them the opportunity to put the events that preceded the current psychotic crisis in chronological order. Whether one is confronting a prepsychotic state, a first episode psychosis, or particular chronic conditions in which the current crisis is just one of a long series of decompensations, putting life events in chronological order provides an initial anchor by which the patient's psyche can reestablish contact with reality.

However, situating time in a spatial dimension is a therapeutic procedure (which I refer to as *spanning*) that is not always possible at the beginning of transactional analytical therapy with the psychotic patient. In general, the more organized and differentiated the Child ego state is, the more chance the spanning process has of being achievable from the early days of the therapy. This is particularly evident in work with paranoid subjects when a distinction between internal parental preobjects and objects (P_{1+} and P_{1-}) is more marked, as evidenced by the transference and countertransference dynamics within the analytic and extra-analytic process (see Chapter 4).

For example, John was convinced that his thoughts were being controlled by his neighbors. He knew this because of the way the pictures in his living room regularly became "crooked." This was proof for him that his neighbors were using ultrasound to interfere with his mind.

(P = Patient, T = Therapist)

P: "I stopped watching TV in the lounge ages ago."

T: "What does the TV have to do with it?"

P: "Because when I sat on the sofa watching the TV, the ultrasound waves passed through the wall where the sofa is and controlled my brain. It meant I couldn't concentrate. I felt tired and sleepy all the time and couldn't understand what they were saying on the TV any more. Do you understand?"

T: "And that means that you have completely stopped turning on the TV since then?"

P: "Yes, exactly. And in fact, to be able to carry on using the living room sofa, I also had to unplug the cable because I was worried that the neighbors' ultrasound waves would be able to bounce off the screen and continue controlling my thoughts. But without electricity, the screen is as good as dead."

T: "Um, what you're telling me must have made life uncomfortable for you."

P: "Uncomfortable? A beam of ultrasound through the whole lounge and since then my thoughts haven't been clear, they are blurred."

T: "And how do you manage to live with this problem?"

P: "I sleep in the kitchen. It's the only place in the house that isn't in the path of the ultrasound beams."

T: "And how long have you slept in the kitchen?"

P: "Including today, 21 days. Exactly 3 weeks ... nonstop."

T: "I wonder how long you have lived in this house though?"

P: "Ah, that's a good question." (Silence while the patient appears to frown and think.) "Nearly 2 years, yes, it was September 2012 when I moved to Steventon Road. So in September it will be 2 years."

T: "And when you did realize that your neighbors were controlling your thoughts with ultrasound?"

P: "I saw it in the crooked pictures."

T: "Yes, yes, you've explained that already. But when did you notice the position of the pictures?"

P: "Well, I've always known actually that the pictures were never straight. The pictures have always been crooked in this house."

T: "And so how can you tell how long your neighbors have been beaming through ultrasound that you believe has been interfering with your thoughts?"

P: (Silence. Patient has visibly changed. He looks at me, frowning, and asks): "Perhaps you know something? Have you spoken to my neighbors?"

T: "John, I know neither your neighbors nor the house where you live at all."

P: "But you know my address and that means that you know exactly where I live."

T: "John, you have just reminded me of your address. We've only known each other about a month."

P: (He looks at me suspiciously and with irritation and then continues): "The pictures, I'm sure, have always been crooked, and I don't know exactly when I started to think ... to think about the fact that they were crooked because of the ultrasound."

T: "In other words, John, you're telling me that the pictures have been crooked ever since you moved to that house, and that at a certain point you connected the crooked pictures with the presence of ultrasound that came from the neighbors' flat next door, but you continue to say that you had always verified the presence of the ultrasound from the crooked position of the pictures ... do you follow what I mean?"

P: "Yes, yes ... I follow." He looks at me thoughtfully.

T: "What are you thinking about?"

P: "That the neighbors might have been controlling me with ultrasound from the first day I set foot in there! Damn it! I have to get out of this fucking place!"

T: "John, it's very important that you are putting the facts into the order they happened."

P: "Yes, but I've said it's their fault that I don't understand anything any more, I'm losing my mind."

T: "Can I ask you another question, John?"

P: "Yes ... of course."

T: "Has it happened before that you've moved house because you thought that neighbors were interfering with you in some way?"

P: "How do you know?"

T: "Know what?"

P: "That I've also had trouble with other neighbors?"

T: "I'm just following your thoughts and your emotions, John, and the events in the order they happened. I'm just trying to understand how long you've had this problem of interference by your neighbors, and perhaps by other people as well."

P: "Well, yes, it's happened before. I left another house after being there only 6 months before moving to Steventon Road."

T: "Is there any chance, John, even remotely, that the problem isn't to do with this or that house, these or those neighbors, but that perhaps there is something within you that doesn't let you live in peace?"

P: "No. Absolutely not. For me the problem is other people. But my neighbors more than anyone."

T: "You're being very honest. For that reason, in order to have this therapy together, it would be useful if you could bear in mind that I too could be seen by you, sooner or later, to be a problem, but I don't want to end up like your neighbors, do you understand?"

P: He stares at me and adds, "Yes, I need to remember that you're here to help me so that I don't lose it."

The case of John suggests that, with appropriate guidance, paranoid individuals are often "lucid" when providing details of important events that preceded the crisis, some of which, however, become quickly infused with delusional meaning triggering in these individuals a major concern until they feel that their own psychic and even physical integrity are at risk. Examining events in terms of a time framework within which it is possible to move around as if in a space of physical time (span)—from past to present up to the future and vice versa—allows the therapist to move the analysis forward in a more or less systematic way through the use of therapeutic techniques aimed at both decontamination and deconfusion of the Child (Berne, 1975a [1961], 1977 [1966]).

In cases of fragmentary psychosis, on the other hand, in which a bodily and nonverbal register of the person's experience predominates, the therapist is inevitably confronted with the early and protomental states of the patient's self. In these cases, spanning is postponed until later in the analysis. Initially it is more helpful to focus primarily on creating the best conditions within the therapeutic setting for containing the emerging bodily-emotional experiences, which can be (as described earlier) destabilizing both for the patient and the therapist. Medication in such cases can help to reduce psychotic anguish, although it is best to use it in such a way as to avoid extinguishing the often polysensory quality of the experiences of fragmentation that torment the individual and fracture his or her ego. In such situations, analysts often have to undergo a bodily-emotional metamorphosis themselves, becoming an active recipient of almost indescribable and highly emotional relational experiences that are endowed with a heightened sense of psychic as well as physical reality.

Through the recovery of the spatial dimension of time—or, practically speaking, through joining up events by means of a "first," a "now," and a "then"—patients can develop awareness of their own history, the history of their own thoughts, emotions, fantasies, bodily-emotional states, and actions relating back to a traumatic event (i.e., an existential discontinuity) (Winnicott, 1990 [1986]) that feeds into the experience of their own self. Before constructing a basis for a future reediting of their own psychobiography, spanning allows these patients to develop awareness of their own real-life experiences, or those lived as such by their "real" self. As Merleau-Ponty (1986 [1945]) neatly said, "We must understand time as the subject and the subject as time" (p. 422).

In the end, it is through the process of spanning that the therapist helps these patients to become aware and hopefully thereby to fulfill their primary needs: to be seen, heard, and accepted as human beings who are able to think, feel, take action, and act responsibly, the latter understood as the capacity, conscious or not, to continue to answer for their own destiny, despite their mental suffering, by the deliberate exertion of their own will.

Situating time in place or context

The process of contextualization is aimed at placing a specific experiential event, recent or past, narrated by the psychotic individual, within an active sociorelational context, imbued by the patient with significant emotional value.

(P = Patient, T = Therapist)

P: "I got lost at university, yes, got lost right from the start."

T: "When you say 'got lost,' Alice, do you mean 'got confused'?"

P: "Yes ... No ... I mean 'lost,' do you understand? Lost. Have you ever been lost somewhere?" said with irritation. (A pause. I wait for more.) "I got lost in the halls of the Alma Mater"... (and then continues to murmur), "Alma Mater ... Alma Mater ... Alma Mater."

T: "Do you mean the sense of feeling controlled by someone else perhaps started there, in Bologna, while you were at university?"

P: "Yes, I really think so ... (long pause) ... I studied, studied, studied day and night, I did ... but I never took an exam ... I was terrified of exams ... I was terrified of this damned 'mummy university.'"

As this short excerpt shows, in cases of paranoid psychosis with a more organized ego, among the factors that precipitate a breakdown is often a significant relational fracture that the person is able to describe, although he or she may interpret the meaning in a delusional way: for example, separation from the nuclear family to move to a new city, the inability to take a university exam, a dispute with a family member or employer, the end of a romantic relationship or long-standing friendship, and so on.

I was struck by the imaginative significance of the words Alice used to refer to her first contact with the university (the Alma Mater Studiorum—Università di Bologna). She described it in a few words as a sort of "cursed" relationship with a new "Alma Mater," which literally means "nurturing mother." Alice's existential experience was emblematic for me because it clarified how, although the context may differ, paranoid schizophrenic individuals on the edge of psychotic crisis come up forcibly against social representations of their own internal Parent or, rather, that particular real person or normative institution able to reflect the primary image of parental authority (*imago parentis*) that was excluded early in their development. These are, in other words, social-relational situations that introduce to the person a "new" Other from the world of adults, an experience that harks back powerfully and traumatically to emotional experiences fiercely fueled inside those primary object and preobject relationships with the big parental Other of his or her infancy (P_1 and P_0). This "dramatic conjunction," which Lacan talks about (1977 [1958]), is the point of origin of the psychosis, which fuses together the present with the individual's past.

The paranoid patient's narrative, therefore, centers on this relational drama, an unforeseen harbinger of unconscious meanings that may not have been repressed (because they are attached on an unconscious level to presymbolic and protomental experiences of development) and that are not yet conscious but which will be coconstructed in the present by the patient and the therapist within the analytic relationship.

In cases of psychotic onset or in paucisymptomatic forms of schizophrenia—for example, in which a bodily-dissociative phenomenology predominates with a more pervasive egoic fragmentation—it is almost never possible to find, at least at the outset, a clear precipitating event. This is the case regardless of how involved the patient's family is, as if the contact with the analyst is the only recognizable, relational event with the ability to trigger the psychotic crisis. When analytic therapy is not the trigger, other relational situations, even those that appear fairly innocuous, can bring about the person's deterioration into active psychosis: for example, one or more visits to the family doctor (e.g., for alleged somatic complaints), one or more consultations with the educational or occupational psychologist, meeting with a spiritual guide, and so on.

A fairly common situation encountered in clinical practice—particularly for those working with people having their first psychotic episode or who are considered at high risk of transition to psychosis—is meeting patients who are young, still adolescent or on the threshold of adulthood, whose source of worry and anguish is essentially their own body. It is not unusual to encounter patients going through puberty who describe concerns about their own self-image, complain of psychosomatic experiences, present symptoms of actual body dysmorphia, have difficulty defining themselves in terms of their own gender identity (male, female, etc.), exhibit unusual behavior around food, or sometimes show the warning signs of an underlying eating disorder and even resort to plastic surgery, convinced they are correcting supposed somatic imperfections. Although this kind of physical malaise can appear to a non-psychotic person to be a serious defect and even as a worrying danger with regard to their physical health, for schizophrenics these experiences of anguish are blown up into a powerful threat to the sense of their own identity. This brings the individual back to the more fundamental questions of "Who am I?" and "Who are you?" and "Whose body is this?"

In other words, for some prepsychotic individuals, as well as those who are experiencing an actual psychotic breakdown, the theater in which the transference dramas of their existence are played out returns to being—as in earliest infancy—the body itself. And this occurs also because of important somatic changes, including neurodevelopmental and hormonal ones, that are typical of adolescence and early adulthood and that happen to be regulated by a more pressing biological, rather than merely existential, clock.

(P = Patient, T = Therapist)

P: "You haven't noticed anything yet?"

T: "Noticed what?"

P: "My jaw, down here, perhaps you can't see it. … It clicks, like a cog … up and down … up and down …" (Tentatively touches himself on the chin with two fingers, slowly opening and shutting his mouth.)

T: (I try as best I can to put forward a checklist as a doctor might and ask): "From what I know, you don't take medication that might cause any of the problems you're talking about. Do you have trouble chewing, or swallowing, or do you suffer from migraine at all?"

P: "No, no, my GP has ruled out a physical problem."

T: "Um, but nevertheless, Chris, you continue to feel something strange in your jaw."

P: "It's stone. … Do you feel it?" (He touches himself a number of times on the chin and, scared, adds, articulating every single word) "It is cold and hard like stone."

Chris's anguish is about the finiteness of his own ego, anguish linked to the perception of cold, petrified, almost dead parts of his own being. The psychotic person's psychological ego becomes in this scenario a bodily presence, hard like stone. And like stone, the psychotic ego, revealing its own fissures through the embodiment of old tensions, historical stressors, and even past relational traumas, returns to being susceptible still to new pressures and possible fractures. But it is precisely the question "Do you feel it?"—which is "Touch! Feel what I've become!" which is "Who am I now?"—that reveals Chris's desperate appeal to the Other, seeking repair, seeking a new organization of self-experience. For Chris, this appeal is distressing because he feels his own psychological ego transmigrating (or passing through) his own body (in this case his jaw) and, in this passing through, (trans)passing away at both a psychological and bodily level of experience. From this then arises the almost ineffable anguish of existential annihilation through petrification and subsequent shattering. However, this split also opens the way to projection, enabling bodily transference. The psychotic ego thus finds the opening and the impetus toward another body, another Other (in this case the therapist).

For individuals such as Chris, this bodily identification brings the ego into contact with the psyche's earliest mental experiences, which are rooted not only in the postnatal period but back in intrauterine experience. These fundamentally establish the nesting of one's own ego in the Other's body and the nesting of the Other in one's own body ego. This indivisible union, this

119

"unrepresentable" as the origin of psychological life, is the incarnate truth as suffered by psychotic individuals. For them, coming up against the boundaries of their own body, acknowledging its physical finiteness, means to (re)feel the disturbing experience of an original insufficiency, of being as a result of the Other, of being for the Other and, ultimately, despite the Other.

Thus, within the body there is again anguish for the Other, an original Other whom the psychotic person has deemed not "good enough," an Other who is intrusive and symbiotic (in some unfortunate cases, even abusive) or actually absent and inaccessible on a bodily-emotional level. This is an Other from whom it has not been possible to separate or individuate without having to resort to fragmentary dissociation, thereby displacing one's own nuclear self elsewhere. This "elsewhere," as in the case of Abena (see Chapter 4) or in Chris's case just described, becomes in these patients' narratives their own body or, more often, a part of it such as a sense organ, a sphincter, a narrower internal organ such as the stomach, the trachea, a specific side of the head, a musculoskeletal articulation, and so on. But this "elsewhere" for which the psychotic yearns is also the body-Other, or an alter ego in flesh and blood—including the analyst—in the tentative hope that it might be able to serve as a new subsidiary body-ego for the patient, containing the anguish of fragmentation and reorganizing the experience of the person's bodily self in its most basic forms of existence.

This preverbal context of existence of the patient in relation to the analyst represents nothing less than the reediting in the analytic setting of the primal protocol. The analytic work with psychotic individuals inevitably results in the (re)discovery of the fundamental role, for the progression of the analysis itself, of the analyst's protocol experiences as they are called on to be an integral part of a bodily setting lived with the patient. It is within this inter-bodily setting that the subsequent and sometimes concurrent process of corporealization described in the next section is possible.

Honoring the present (or giving space to present time)

From a psychodynamic perspective on the therapeutic setting, maintaining clear spatiotemporal boundaries helps to make the analytic space a special container within which the analytic experience can unfold. My own clinical experience with psychotic patients, even those who are quite young—whether on an acute psychiatric ward or in an intensive home treatment setting, including multidisciplinary work under the careful supervision of clinicians who are experts at looking after people in their first manifestation of a schizophrenic psychosis—has allowed me to dedicate to such patients longer and more intensive sessions of transactional analysis than those conventionally offered in psychotherapy contracts (as in outpatient clinics both in the public and private sectors).

This way of working, which produced a seminal work on the transactional analytic psychopathology of schizophrenic psychoses (Mellacqua, 2014), has found an almost unique but powerful resonance in the ideas developed by Bollas (2013) in his book *Catch them before they fall: The psychoanalysis of breakdown*. In it he daringly asserts that "more than anything, the patient who is breaking down needs time" (p. 75). I add "daringly" because in the normal analytic setting, the traditional psychoanalyst, and also the transactional analyst—albeit with different lengths and frequency of sessions per week and depending on whether the analytic work is with a group or an individual—have spaces and times that are fairly standardized.

The time Bollas talks about is primarily the time of the person and, more particularly, the time of the psychotic individual, which is an eternally present time where "the past is a dream," "the future exists only as a black hole," and "the self tries to live in a perpetual waking present" (Bollas, 2013, p. 78).

From this point—which is the point of the patient's subjectivity, the point at which, according to Berne, the Child expresses itself phenomenologically— the analytic setting needs to undergo a temporal distortion so that more space (and therefore more chronological time) can be given to the subjective time of the psychotic patient. By "honoring the present," I mean intentionally expanding the temporal space (time span) conventionally given to the time of an analytic session. This would allow extending it, for example, to many hours, or to different hours distributed through the course of the same day, or, for example in Bollas's (2013, 2015) experience, filling an entire day or being repeated over a number of consecutive days. Likewise, the analytic work can also be restricted and broken down into many daily sessions of a quarter or half an hour (as often happens in hospital or during longer hospitalizations, for example, in rehabilitation or forensic settings).

Obviously, such a marked distortion of the analytic setting necessarily requires extraordinary flexibility on the part of the therapist as well as on the part of the organization for which he or she works, and for many it is neither practical nor possible.

However, it is this valuable opportunity to open up the analytic setting to the subjectivity of psychotic patients that enables not only the quick reparation of the experiential fractures in their ego but also to facilitate joint attention to their spatial alignment and temporal consolidation, which ultimately encourages the integration of self-experience.

References

Berne, E. (1975a). *Transactional analysis in psychotherapy: A systematic individual and social psychiatry*. London: Souvenir Press. (Original work published 1961)

Berne, E. (1975b). *What do you say after you say hello? The psychology of human destiny*. London: Corgi. (Original work published 1972)

Berne, E. (1977). *Principles of group treatment*. New York: Grove Press. (Original work published 1966)

Bollas, C. (1987). *The shadow of the object: Psychoanalysis of the unthought known*. New York, NY: Columbia University Press.

Bollas, C. (2002). What is this thing called self? In C. Bollas, *Cracking up: The work of unconscious experience* (pp. 146–179). London: Routledge. (Original work published 1995)

Bollas, C. (2006). Aspects of self experiencing. In C. Bollas, *Being a character: Psychoanalysis and self experience* (pp. 11–32). London: Routledge. (Original work published 1992)

Bollas, C. (2013). *Catch them before they fall: The psychoanalysis of breakdown*. London: Routledge.

Bollas, C. (2015). *When the sun bursts: The enigma of schizophrenia*. New Haven, CT: Yale University Press.

Cornell, W. F. (2015). *Somatic experience in psychoanalysis and psychotherapy: In the expressive language of the living*. London: Routledge.

Federn, P. (1953). *Ego psychology and the psychoses*. London: Imago Publishing. (Original work published 1952)

Lacan, J. (1977). On a question prior to any possible treatment of psychosis. In J. Lacan, J. A. Miller (Ed.), *Écrits: The first complete edition in English* (B. Fink, Trans.). New York, NY: Norton. (Original work published 1958)

Mellacqua, Z. (2014). Beyond symbiosis: The role of primal exclusion in schizophrenic psychosis. *Transactional Analysis Journal*, 44, 8–30.

Merleau-Ponty, M. (1986). *The phenomenology of perception* (C. Smith, Trans.). London: Routledge & Kegan Paul. (Original work published 1945)

Winnicott, D. W. (1965). *The maturational processes and the facilitating environment: Studies in a theory of emotional development*. Madison, CT: International Universities Press.

Winnicott, D. W. (1990). *Home is where we start from: Essays by a psychoanalyst*. London: Penguin Book. (Original work published 1986)

6

THE BODY IN ACTION

Protocol analysis in schizophrenia

Reality sensing

If *reality testing* is the task par excellence of the Adult ego state, the experience of the real through the senses—what I refer to as *reality sensing*—is the Child's prerogative. The Child's primary concern is not the verbal formulation of transmissible meanings but the lived-in organization of the self's experience.

When working with psychotic patients, the first thing to do is to support this process of polysensory attunement to reality (including the reality of one's own body) through which these individuals can (re)organize their self-experience and experience of others and the external world within the boundaries of sensoriality. Garfield (2009 [2005]) translated this as applied in analytic work with psychotic patients when he wrote, "The analyst ... serves as the patient's own missing eyes, ears and hands. The therapist becomes, in some respects, a living part of the patient's experience" (p. ix).

It is, therefore, through the (re)discovery of the limits of one's own senses that it becomes possible for the nuclear self to inhabit an egoic space of which it is not master because of the inescapably interbodily and relational nature of the ego. Through analysis, psychotic individuals usually end up in the disturbing position of experiencing the limitations of their own senses while they are simultaneously wrestling with the sense and meanings that they can build in relation to their limits (also bodily). In this proposal, I distinguish the *sensorial limit*, understood as a biologically mediated threshold above which one forms experiences of something and someone, from a *personal boundary*, understood as a relationally mediated threshold above which that something or someone becomes evident to me as other-than-me.

For individuals who are mentally well, the discovery of the boundaries of their own ego can occur through repeated, sensorial contacts (or impacts) with the Other. This is an Other who does not intrude or completely withdraw from the relationship but who comes and goes unceasingly despite these contacts, an Other who generously allows itself to be deformed and transformed by the individual, thereby reciprocally supporting its own

123

deformation and transformation as a person. The concept of personal boundary thus retains the trace left by the Other on the person's own ego. In other words, the ego boundary is as it is because it preserves the memory of the historical-Other. The challenge for contemporary transactional analysis in work with psychotic patients is to recover the memory of the historical Other not primarily in the patients' mind but in their body, in their poly-sensoriality—in their gestures, movements, primal images, and dreams—and then to allow them to coshape a new perception of the self, of the current-Other and the world, in the present reality of the therapeutic and extra-therapeutic relationship.

Touching

The psychological processes that are active in the very early stages of an individual's psychophysical development—grouped together under the term *primary process* by Freud (1958a [1911]) and picked up again by Berne (1975b [1972]) as the redolent image of *tissue experiences* of the self—are inseparable from the body and are spread over the body's surface, including the skin, and into the musculature. In this way, the emerging ego becomes, on the one hand, defined and, on the other, functionally activated by this bodily inter-face, this tissue limen that separates, while also organizing, the internal psy-chic world from external reality, the self from the other-than-self. For the double structure of the skin's system—also anatomically separated into dermis (deep part) and epidermis (surface part)—the development of a func-tioning *skin-Ego* (Anzieu, 1989) cannot occur without mutual exchanges with the Other, an Other that from the beginning of bodily and mental life is per-ceived at a tissue level as a skin-Other.

Tactile transactions during the neonatal and infancy period between infant and primary caregiver(s) promote, on the one hand, nonconscious inter-nalization of the tissue extension of the Other (P_0) and, on the other, a pre-egotization of interbody preobject states (C_0)—even prenatally—merging into a largely nonconscious representation of an interbodily nuclear self (A_0). Subsequent tactile exchanges—cosupported by polysensory (e.g., visual, oral, and olfactory) experiences—with good enough primary reference figures will allow the infant to discover himself or herself as a bodily-self with its own three-dimensionality (C_1). This is the Somatic Child in Woollams and Brown's (1978) sense as distinct from a bodily-Other that can be internalized as a primal representation (primal imago) of a primary object relationship (P_1).

These profound early transactions between the child and his or her care-givers also form the subsymbolic basis (Bucci, 1997, 2008, 2011)—simulta-neously bodily and (proto)mental (Bion, 1961)—of the nuclear experience of the self or the script protocol (Berne, 1975a [1961], 1975b [1972], 1977b [1966]). From this protocol, the individual, continuing to use a logical paral-lelism in the terminology of Bucci (1997), will be able to organize a more articulated "symbolic nonverbal" narrative—provided by primal images, the palimpsest, and dream activity—and a "verbal symbolic" narrative (i.e., the script) of the experience of the self, others, and life in general.

As a transactional analyst who works mainly in clinical practice and who was born, raised, and in large part professionally trained in the south of Italy, I regularly touch my patients. The way I do this, particularly during psychotherapy, is usually with a handshake—or at least by offering the patient the option of a handshake—at the end of each session. There have been instances in which, because I am not trained in body psychotherapy, this has led to such catastrophic sessions methodologically speaking that the quality of the therapeutic relationship has been compromised, or, in some cases, the patient has left therapy or a number of supervision sessions have been required.

Nevertheless, because of my intensive work with psychotic patients and many years of valuable supervision, I have learned "on my skin" to recognize the importance of bodily transactions through touch in the analytic setting as well as in the medical-psychiatric setting (whether in the hospital or a patient's home). I believe I have naturally (re)discovered the reality of my own living body, particularly as a result of my regular "contact" with psychotic patients. As a result, as a therapist I am more focused on the body than I was during my training in psychiatry and transactional analysis. I have found increasing acknowledgment and support for this personal "body orientation" in my clinical practice from reading the important work of authors such as Bick (1968, 2002 [1986]), Anzieu (1989), McDougall (1989, 1995), Resnik (2001 [1972], 2002 [1986], 2005, 2007 [1982]), Benedetti (1997 [1992]), Bloom (2006), and, more recently, Lemma (2015), Cornell (2015), and Bollas (2015).

In particular, Cornell (2015) wrote that the use of the body in therapy is not necessarily synonymous with physical contact between therapist and patient. When one or more tactile experiences occur in the therapeutic setting—just as happens with words—they can be expressed, understood, and exchanged in different ways and on different relationship levels, thereby forming themselves into actual bodily transactions. This is particularly crucial in therapeutic work with patients at the onset of a schizophrenic psychosis, when a special sensibility about the patient's tactile experiences—analytic and extra-analytic—is required by the therapist.

In my clinical experience, the approach to the psychotic patient's tactile experiences is either phenomenological (i.e., aimed at accepting subjective bodily experience as the patient (re)lives them in the present) or analytical (i.e., aimed at exploring the meanings of these bodily experiences as they are (re)constructed and coconstructed in the current therapeutic relationship). This is done with awareness of the patient's relationship history (also inter-bodily) with significant others from his or her past.

Regarding the intervention of intentional physical touching during an analytic session, this is best preceded by letting the patient know in advance and undertaking it with his or her agreement. However, I have used this procedure only rarely in my clinical work with psychotic patients and not without creating therapeutic rapport with the individual first.

One possible scenario occurs when a patient is so polarized in relation to his or her actual bodily experiences that all access to a symbolic register based on primal images (such as to a more definite verbal and cognitive dimension) is foreclosed. The therapist is then inevitably invited by the patient to relate on an extraverbal and protomental level.

For example, I met Sally a few hours after her first admission onto the ward. She was in her twenties and experiencing her first psychotic breakdown. Her housemate, a fellow student, had called the emergency services because she had noticed a progressive psychological deterioration in Sally. She had seemed increasingly distracted, preoccupied, and over recent days, had withdrawn into her bedroom, become mute, and stopped eating and caring for herself. Sally's parents were on holiday in Spain when she was hospitalized.

In her hospital room, because of her rather bizarre behavior Sally attracted the attention and interest of a large group of professionals. When I saw her alone for the first time in her room, I was not able to engage her in verbal communication. Sally was barefoot, had a vacant look, and was staring into space with her head slightly bowed and allowed almost to fall diagonally in front of her; she appeared to ignore what was going on around her, who was with her at the moment, and what was being said to her. Sally was absorbed in something very personal, not easy to see or understand, but her body was not still. Merleau-Ponty (1986 [1945]) noted how the body comes to "symbolize existence because it realizes it and is its actuality" (p. 164).

Sally spent many hours tracing with small, quick steps the exact perimeter of her room, except for one side of it, an invisible side, but also immediately obvious to me, inasmuch as it was a side regularly traced by her movement in the same place. Sally's psyche seemed like a body in movement, revealing doggedly regular trajectories as if to frame the invisible, the inexpressible, the ungraspable. I came to doubt whether Sally was even aware of the passing of time. She did not have aids such as a watch or mobile phone that could tell her the time or date. In that room, in semidarkness, it seemed that she was creating new coordinates of space and time that were not immediately obvious to me. Paradoxically, what I actually started to feel was a rising sense of inertia, as if everything in that room happened by inertia, as if even I had arrived there by inertia, and the world in there was all equal, recursive, flat, always the same. After nearly half an hour of being there, I became aware of a kind of "mental inebriation" mixed with a growing anguish.

Not perceiving anything threatening in Sally's behavior, it occurred to me to physically enter the perimeter of "her" room. I did this in silence, occupying a little area right in the middle of her perimeter of steps, not far from the bed. Some minutes passed. Neither of us said a word. At a certain point, I made as if to leave, and only then did she break out of her perimeter and come to me as if she was upset by my going. I stopped, continuing to observe her behavior. She came close to me until she bumped gently against my hip. Then, for the first time since I entered her room, she lifted her head and made fleeting eye contact with me. With this unconscious cointentionality, a way of communicating had been initiated, one made of gestures, actions, and now also of looks between me and Sally.

Sally spent almost four months in the hospital and reluctantly accepted a low dose of antipsychotic medication. Our meetings continued, and after nearly two weeks I became the target of erotic projections in which Sally strenuously maintained that she had had sex with me. At a certain point, she even claimed that she was expecting a son, "our son." For months I had to engage in supervision in order to contain and make sense of the patient's bodily transference while maintaining an attitude of curiosity still centered on the bodily experience of us both.

In the wake of the brief but intense psychotherapeutic work with Sally, which went on for around two years in an outpatient capacity, my clinical experience with these patients, especially at the onset of their psychosis, led me to believe that every bodily transaction—and above all those based on direct physical contact—ideally needs to be properly thought out in advance by the therapist. This is for two reasons, which, given the type of suffering experienced by these individuals, have important ethical implications. On the one hand, many of these patients present with a polytraumatic history (including actual physical and even sexual abuse). On the other, for some of these patients, their body has become, from earliest infancy and then into puberty, the main arena for the expression of both relational dynamics with symbiotic value (not necessarily abusive) and dramatic deprivation of inter-human contact with primary caregivers. In either case, the risk with psychotic patients who are "imprisoned" in their body is of exposing them, through direct physical contact, to bodily (re)traumatization. This can lead them back to primitive states of psychophysical dependence (regression and fusion) in the absence of clear, verbalizable material.

Nevertheless, the therapeutic element in work involving physical "con-tact-ing" consists of the fact that this process often leads schizophrenic patients to "contact" intense emotional states, both actual and historical, that necessarily require consensual emotional holding (as explained in the following section on "emotional containment"). From this comes the possibility of forming a connection between somatic experiences and comprehensible emotional states but within a new interbodily relationship (which I refer to as *somatic-affective bridging*).

Looking and primal imaging

From the origins of our relational life, the ineffable trading of looks between mother, father (or primary caregivers), and their newborn baby is what allows the nuclear self to grow as a visible object for the Other and as a subject who "regards" the Other. This consideration guides the following observations: in nearly normal development, one cannot see oneself without first watching an Other, or be or feel oneself to be seen without first being watched by an Other, or feel acknowledged and loved without the regard of an Other. This means that looking is propedeutic to reflection and therefore to intimacy and mutual recognition (also understood as Bernean OK-ness) between individuals who come to recognize each other as unique and unrepeatable subjects. Grounding the role of reflection in the analytic process, Winnicott (1971) made clear how psychotherapy is

> a complex derivative of the face that reflects what is there to be seen. I like to think of my work this way, and to think that if I do this well enough the patient will find his or her own self, and will be able to exist and to feel real.
>
> (p. 117)

The analytic relationship with psychotic patients, even more than with other individuals, requires that the best possible conditions in the physical setting be maintained in order to ensure and encourage this mutual mirroring between analyst and patient. In practical terms, this translates as the systematic use, although not necessarily exclusively, of chairs or sofas arranged opposite each other or in a circle (as in a group setting) rather than a couch (with its obvious psychoanalytic overtones). This methodological assumption, which is particularly close to Berne's (1977b [1966]) thoughts on the matter, maintains that eye contact is another door that opens into the representational internal world (unconscious and nonconscious) of both the patient and the analyst. In other words, because the exchange of looks is, along with the first tissue and polysensory experiences, the basis of the experience of the Child ego state—that is, of an infantile self that historically shapes itself in relation to a significant other(s)—bodily transactions that are phenomenologically observable via eye contact between therapist and psychotic patient form a different powerful aspect of transference and countertransference. As such, they contribute useful information for subsequent analytic work based on the coconstruction of interpretative hypotheses.

In clinical practice, psychotic individuals' level of alienation is ascertainable from both the direction their eyes are looking as well the ability of their gaze to act (or not) as a *social mirror* in relation to the other, including the therapist. The psychotic's gaze is frequently referred to as a "fixed look," "empty look," "sullen look," "averted look," and even "absent look." This reflects how the facial register conveys more than words are able to in the schizophrenic experience.

As mentioned earlier, Berne himself (1975a [1961]) used a visual metaphor, which I have retained and expanded to describe the process of Parent exclusion experienced like a "one-way glass" (p. 66). This describes in a visually meaningful way the subjective experience of the psychotic person with respect to the Other (including the therapist) in terms of alternately being on this and that side of the "one-way glass," able to act either as eye, lens, or screen (as in paranoia), on the one hand, or as filter, mask, and even protective shield (as in fragmentary schizophrenias), on the other.

In both cases, the monodirectionality of the "gaze" from one part of the ego to another (P_1 toward C_1) and vice versa (C_1 toward P_1) is translated in the psychotic individual into a monodirectional look toward and from the therapist within the analytic setting. The therapist's task is to resolve this *visual disattunement* as (re)presented within the analytic relationship so that the patient can progressively regain the view of the Other, even if this is painful and in some cases even blinding, through the eyes, and therefore through the view, of the therapist. For these reasons, the patient's reappropriation of his or her *visual ability* represents a process that is both interbodily and relational. This process allows the patient's ego to expand its feeling of reality and thereby have access to a new awareness of self and Other through the real and actual relationship with the therapist. This sensory expansion of the ego, through the eyes, reactivates bodily-emotional states associated with early phases of psychological development (Bion, 1984 [1967]) with potentially progressive, and not necessarily regressive, implications for the psychotic individual's sense of identity. This seems to be true not only in work with adult psychotics but also in certain forms of adolescent psychotic breakdown (Lombardi & Pola, 2010).

For this reason, the beginning of analytic therapy can act as a trigger that unleashes in the person a surge of deep existential pain—both bodily and mental—mixed with the hate and anguish that accompany the start of "perceiving" himself or herself as fragile without the Other and, at the same time, alone and needing the Other. French philosopher Jean Paul Sartre (1992 [1943]) encapsulated this disturbing quality of the Other's gaze—simultaneously the basis of the individual's identity—when he wrote, "The Other looks at me and as such holds the secret of my being, he knows what I am. Thus the profound meaning of my being is outside of me" (p. 363).

In the case of paranoid schizophrenia, for example, the person feels constantly under the persecutory scrutiny of an Other who often disappears from view: now an opaque Other who can see but cannot be seen (from which comes Berne's idea of exclusion as *one-way glass*, Berne, 1975a [1961], p. 66), now a ubiquitous Other whose presence is multiplied through the eyes of everyone else (including the therapist).

Returning to the case of Mr Blake, discussed in Chapter 4, he used to come to our psychotherapy sessions always wearing a pair of black sunglasses with very dark lenses. Now it is not the case that the sun never shines in London, but sunny days there are infrequent enough that not many people wear sunglasses even outside the therapy room. But Mr Blake was accustomed to putting on his sunglasses every time he left the house, day or night.

(P = Patient, T = Therapist)

T: "I can see that yours has become such a habit that you put on your sunglasses almost automatically when you leave the house."

The patient stays silent, keeping his head directed toward me.

T: "What I'm wondering ..."

On the patient's face I see the ghost of a smile as he adds, "Where are you going with this, doctor?"

T: "Well, I find it unusual for someone to wear a pair of such dark sunglasses, at least in this room."

P: "My eyes are used to the dark now. I find the light in here very intense. Everything is very strong here and aggressive for me."

T: "Are you saying that perhaps I am very intense for you? That you feel 'attacked' by me in these sessions?"

He smiles placidly. Then in a sudden motion he takes off his glasses, holding them tightly in his fist, and, looking thoughtful, tells me, "There is something strange in here!"

I stay still. I allow a moment of silence. And then calmly I say to him, "Up to now I have found it unusual and strange, if you like, that you wear dark glasses during therapy."

He smiles oddly while just as suddenly lifting the glasses to his face to put them back on.

T: "It is strange for me, Mr Blake, not to be able to look you directly in the eye. It is strange to feel myself seen by you, almost as if you are constantly scrutinizing me, without being able to see your expression, to understand what you are thinking or what you are feeling while you're talking to me ... this is basically why I feel uncomfortable."

After a moment of silence, he says to me, "Yes," touching himself nervously on the nose. Then he adds, "Just think, doctor: I feel like that every day." Mr Blake encountered early on pain connected with the intrusivity as well as the inscrutability of his primary Other's gaze, in particular in the preobject and object relationship with his maternal figure. Paradoxically, the fact that he wore the glasses allowed me to experiment with his own subjective position in relation to others. Our therapy sessions, instead, shone a light, as it were, directly on his eyes. He did not like to reveal them for fear of once again being invaded and blinded by the impenetrability of the Other and, at the same time, because of the terror of seeing a "different" reality from that of his infancy, namely, one seen with different eyes and in a new light.

Mr Blake's condition shows, moreover, how the paranoid solution that such individuals reach for reasons of psychophysical survival during their early developmental years then becomes an obstacle to the progression of their own self's sense of identity, the expansion of which involves the reinclusion of the excluded primary Other. The persecutory state of the paranoid individual can even culminate in real demonstrations of hate toward the Other (including the therapist)—with explosive verbal and sometimes physical aggression, as if trying to escape the relationship—when the person feels the relationship with the therapist to be particularly intense, at times even outrageous on a moral level and threatening on a bodily-emotional level.

On the other hand, in dissociative or fragmentary schizophrenias, avoiding the gaze of the other while not avoiding his or her presence, or "spying" on the other when he or she is not watching, can enable the psychotic to evade the existential pain associated with the discovery of his or her own fragility and loneliness, both connected to the realization of his or her separateness from the other (including the therapist).

For example, Anisha was in her forties, of Indian origin, and had been living in the Camberwell area for 10 years in a small flat that she owned. She had been known to the local psychiatric services for a little less than a decade as having a paucisymptomatic form of schizophrenia corresponding largely to the nosographic criteria for schizophrenia simplex. She was referred to our team for an intensive psychiatric home treatment intervention by her psychiatrist, who had, in turn, been approached by her grandchildren after they noticed a deterioration in her psychological state. Anisha's family had reported to the general practitioner that she was no longer answering the phone, had, of her own volition, stopped her medications, was neglecting her domestic and personal hygiene, and had often been spotted around her area walking long distances on foot pulling a trolley that, apart from anything else, was very heavy.

With no small reluctance, and faced otherwise with the likelihood of compulsory admission to a psychiatric ward, the patient had voluntarily accepted domiciliary care by the Lambeth home treatment team for which I worked as a psychiatrist. I was quickly able to begin building a therapeutic relationship with Anisha, and we agreed on daily home visits. The main difficulty I encountered was her general attitude to our meetings: she allowed me (and in the evening the nurses) access to her house, but she would exchange only a few words, which would then be followed by a long silence. This was repeated daily up to the moment of saying goodbye shortly before I left. She also refused all pharmacological treatment and simple medical testing, such as a blood test or measuring her blood pressure.

This was a particularly arduous situation for the whole team because it was almost impossible to maintain verbal communication with Anisha. Although I also felt on several occasions a sense of impotence and almost an inability to think during my meetings with her, something caught my attention from the beginning: her gaze, or rather, the absence of her gaze. From the moment she opened her front door to let me in, her face was constantly turned toward the floor. Another oddity was the trolley she pulled around; it was of medium size and black, its heavy weight evident from the noise the wheels made when effortfully dragged across the ground under Anisha's vigorous thrusting. In addition, the welcome into her house had a sort of ritual to it: first I would hear the noise of the trolley drawing near to the door, then the door would be opened with the key accompanied by a low "hello" said in an American accent, then we would walk toward the living room going through a second door that was also locked with a key. She walked backward, always dragging the trolley while she shut both doors behind us. Finally, she would invite me to sit on the one free armchair opposite hers in the living room. Then silence. We were also in semidarkness, although the room was somewhat visible.

One day I arrived unassumingly at her house, and after the ritual greeting, I started with, "That photo is very nice, Anisha. Is it of an important ceremony?"

(P = Patient, T = Therapist)

P: "Yes, it was on the occasion of my final thesis on a course at Princeton."

T: "At Princeton? In the United States?"

P: "Yes."

T: "Wow. That's why it immediately struck me that you have an American accent. And what did you study at Princeton?"

P: "A course on Indian literature ... in the department of English and Comparative Studies."

T: "Um, and how did it go?" I tried to ask, with tremulous voice.

P: "You don't believe me, doctor, do you?"

T: "How do you mean, why should I not believe you?"

P: "Dr Stewart laughed in my face when I told him I studied at Princeton."

T: "Um ... it must be said that it's not very common to study at such a prestigious university."

P: "Look over there, near the curtain."

T: "Where?"

P: "This time I'm afraid you'll have to get up and go to the window."
    I get up and cautiously approach the window "Here, you say, on the right?"

P: "Yes, do you see it?"

T: "Wow, this is a bachelor degree certificate!"

P: "Yes," she replies, pleased.

T: "Congratulations Anisha. Your parents must have been proud of you."
    There follows a long pause.

T: "Those are your parents in the photo?"

P: "Which photo? The one with the gown?"

T: "Yes, that one."

P: "No... they are just two colleagues from my course."

T: "Ah, I see. It's just that they seem much older than you."

P: "Yes, they are. A photo of my parents is on the table behind you, on that little table in the corner."
    I try to turn around, a little disoriented. "Where?"

P: "On your right."

T: "Ah, it's right here, I didn't see it."

P: "People look but they don't see."... Another pause and then she adds, "If you turn to your left instead, on that black bookcase, down there."

T: "Yes?"

P: "Can you see it? On the first shelf up from the bottom, there is a book, do you see it?"

T: "Oh yes." I move toward the bookshelf and bend down. "This one here?" while I reach my hand out to grasp the dusty book ... "um *Hungry Stones* by Tagore?"

P: "Yes. Tagore. Do you know him?"

T: "No, well, yes in the sense that I know of Tagore but as a poet, not a writer."

Silence again with her gaze aimed downward. Then she adds, "I don't have much time. I must go back to my studies."

T: "What do you mean? You study?"

P: "Yes, of course. I'm preparing for a new exam."

T: "Ah ... I'm a bit confused ... I thought you had ..."

P: "I am perfecting my literature studies at Princeton."

T: "Ah, I understand," I said hesitatingly.

P: "No, you don't understand. You're only wasting my time."

T: "I'm sorry, I didn't want to annoy you ... I just thought that ... Can I ask what you are currently studying?"

P: "We'll talk about it another time."

She gets up suddenly and decisively grasps the already-raised handle of the trolley, dragging it toward the front door. In that situation, I could only follow Anisha to the door, accepting the fact that I was taking my leave of her and agreeing to see her the following day.

It is clear that during that meeting what I said or, better still, *how* I said it, had ultimately profoundly irritated Anisha to the point where our communication broke down. In fact, something else seemed to have occurred between us that I understood only after having left her house that day. By means of bodily transference, I had unconsciously *lent my eyes* to the patient, allowing her to make me see what she, in a way that was almost omnipotent and con-fusional, wanted me to see, namely precious, somewhat remote, corners of her internal world: the photo showing her at the ceremony with her two course colleagues, her degree certificate, the photo of her parents, and the book by Tagore.

On the other hand, every uncertainty I showed when seeing what she wanted me to see, every slight doubt that crept into my voice about the truth of her account, had in some way shaken the walls of that world, which was imaginary inasmuch as, for more than 20 years, Anisha had felt herself to be an eternal student, still intending to take exams at the prestigious university of Princeton. This experience, which was very private for her, had become a sort of "secret life" that captured her from the inside, distancing her emotionally from the subsequent failures in her real life in social, work, and family contexts. For these reasons, she always directed her gaze elsewhere and always seemed about to leave, to return forever to a world that was, perhaps, the last time she had really felt alive, where she had been satisfied with something or had perhaps been important to someone. My presence thus represented a potential threat to her internal world, to the imaginary existence that protected her from other people (including me), in whose gaze she risked finding reflected her own fragility and profound loneliness.

In contrast, in other situations the eye contact made by psychotic individuals with their therapists is "diverted," with the double meaning of "happy" (able to feel happy themselves as well as to make their interlocutor happy) and "to be directed elsewhere" (from the latin *divertere*, meaning "turn away," blended from *di(s)* and *vertere* "to turn") outside the analytic relationship. This extra-analytic space to which the "diverted" gaze of these psychotic patients returns is, in fact, a space in their mind in which live fragments of visual, and sometimes polysensory, experiences from their past, charged with a strong bodily-emotional energy. These mental images—which are distinct from normal images in the memory because of their perceptual quality and which lead the person immediately back to an object relationship from infancy—were called *primal images* by Berne (1977a [1955], Chapter 4). He also elucidated how primal images presumably also exist in other sensory realms besides the visual (Berne, 1977a [1955], p. 70). In his definition, these appear particularly close to Anzieu's (1989, 1990 [1987]) concept of the *psychic envelope*. They are situated on the boundary between the subsymbolic and the symbolic-nonverbal that Bucci (1997) wrote about. As Berne (1977a [1955]) wrote, "Primal images are presymbolic representations of interpersonal transactions, whose study leads directly into certain important areas of psychopathology" (p. 67).

In clinical practice, psychotic patients can present as absorbed in a kind of internal scene, as if dreaming with their eyes open, which can be linked to stereotypical behaviors such as slight movements of the face and mouth, the appearance of reflexes (e.g., sucking), loss of control over sphincters (anal, urethral), and sometimes saying barely audible words or fragments of phrases.

I will give here a short fragment of my psychotherapeutic work with Miguel, a patient in his twenties with a hebephrenic schizophrenia. He was referred to me by a private psychiatrist following deterioration in his mental state with progressive social isolation, frequent episodes of nocturnal enuresis, and apparently illogical thoughts that had begun some months after the sudden death of his mother from a heart attack. Accompanying him to every session was his aunt, the sister of the patient's mother.

During the first weeks of therapy, which was carried out over two sessions per week, at a certain point in the session I found him particularly immersed in one of his visual hallucinations. At those points, he generally appeared visibly distracted.

(P = Patient, T = Therapist)

P: "Ha ha ... yes ... Ha ha ..." laughing for no apparent reason.

T: "What is funny, Miguel?"

After a moment of silence he gave a quiet laugh: "Ha ha ... yes. Ha ha ..." lifting his arms almost mechanically, which then fell suddenly to dangle at the sides of the chair. He almost didn't seem to notice I was there. His gaze fell absently on something that or someone who seemed to amuse him, as if he was in front of a cinema screen placed somewhere to the right of me.

T: "I'd like to laugh with you," I added in a vaguely amused way.

Instead there followed a new series of smothered laughs, while darting me quick glances, and then I heard him say in a deep voice, almost distracted, "Mickey Mouse ... Ha ha ... Mickey Mouse ..."

T: "Ah Mickey Mouse ... Have I understood you? You're watching Mickey Mouse?"

P: "You're funny ... ha ha ... You make me laugh Mickey Mouse," said this time with a noticeable Portuguese accent, which made the interaction even more diverting.

T: "Ah this is good," I responded, curious, and then added, "So, tell me, how would I be Mickey Mouse?"

P: "Your nose, doctor, sorry, ok? Your nose is like a mouse's."

And while he started laughing uncontrollably, repeatedly wriggling around awkwardly on his chair, he suddenly wet himself, completely involuntarily. I couldn't believe it. But it happened right there in the therapy room. A large stream of incredibly strong-smelling urine started to flow from his trouser leg, creating a particularly wet patch in his crotch area. From that point on in the session, Miguel became visibly anxious, repeatedly apologizing for what had happened, then becoming completely mute and sitting almost paralyzed in his chair, with a fixed gaze turned toward the floor, deeply embarrassed in my presence.

I reassured him a number of times, and we mutually decided to end the session. We promptly asked his aunt for help because she was in the waiting room, and she quickly took him into the bathroom to help him clean himself up. At the behest of his aunt, Miguel turned up to subsequent sessions wearing a pad to avoid any unnecessary repeat of that unfortunate occurrence. Nevertheless, episodes of incontinence continued to be a general feature of future sessions.

During the course of the analysis itself, Miguel was told by his aunt that when he was little, and particularly around the age of five, he was "abandoned" for many hours in his room by his mother and left there to watch TV, often until late at night. His aunt, who regularly visited the house at that time, had found Miguel in his room on a number of occasions with a nappy soaked in urine. Mickey Mouse was his favorite cartoon. In his flat in East London, he had a complete collection of comics about Walt Disney's mouse. Miguel was fiercely possessive of this collection because they were magazines given to him as presents over the years by his mother.

As the sessions went on, we encountered "visions" of Mickey Mouse again and again to the point where it became increasingly clear that those imaginary scenes had infantile antecedents and were in some way connected to the patient's progressive withdrawal into an imaginary internal world that was able to interfere with reality. Those long, perhaps even very long, periods in which Miguel, while still young, was alone and completely neglected, even in his personal needs, were due to the fact that his mother received "many visitors" to the house. At these times she forbade her son to come out of his room, and when Miguel told her he was scared of being by himself for so long, he was angrily told to "be a good boy and play with Mickey Mouse."

Miguel's aunt confirmed that it was probably one of the hardest periods for Miguel and his mother following their arrival in England. Miguel's father had never accepted her pregnancy and left her a few months before Miguel was born. Miguel's mother moved to Reading, not far from London, alone with her son, who had just turned two. Unable to find work, for almost three years Miguel's mother had worked as a prostitute to make a living, and she met her "clients" in the flat where she lived with her son. It was only when her sister arrived that the patient's mother found the impetus to leave the black hole of prostitution and associated alcohol abuse and began to take on small jobs as a cleaning lady for a local company. Miguel, however, had learning disabilities and required a special needs teacher while at primary school. The suspicion that he also was mentally retarded was not subsequently confirmed. The first psychotic symptoms, characterized by hallucinatory phenomena and withdrawal into a fantasy world populated by comic book characters, arose instead around the age of 12, the age from which the start of his psychiatric history dated.

I have described Miguel's story here, first, because it brings powerfully to our attention Berne's initial and exemplary observations on the link between primal images and precise areas of the body that are susceptible to physiological excitation: the so-called "erogenous zones" (Freud, 1958b [1905]), which have been recruited by the ego for *social expression* during infancy. This gives credence, among other things, to the presence of "a deep and persistent infantile quality in object relationships" (Berne, 1977a [1955], p. 67).

During the first phase of therapy with Miguel, I observed how he felt great anguish not only currently because of his mother's death but also because of feelings of rage or even sadness, never expressed, toward her. The uncontrollable release of his urethral sphincter had presumably become for Miguel the preferred channel through which some inexpressible emotions—such as rage and opposition—had found a primary social expression within the object

136

relationship with his mother. This time too, although his mother had permanently abandoned him on the level of reality, his Mickey Mouse allowed him, as in the repeated and traumatic absences of his mother during his infancy, to escape (and this time even deny) the painful experience of the real loss of his parent. Not only that, but the therapy room, like the room of his infancy, risked becoming for Miguel, and for me, a fantasy world in which to take refuge from the psychotic terror of disintegration and psychological annihilation. In fact, I had been recruited omnipotently by Miguel into his internal world in the guise of Mickey Mouse.

It is also useful to observe here how in this state of dissociation from reality, the patient identified omnipotently with Mickey Mouse—"Mickey" and "Miguel" have, apart from anything else, the same root and semantic meaning. At the same time, Miguel massively projected onto me the product of this identification, creating an incessant coming and going of introjection and projection (introjective identification and projective identification). Moreover, the almost-three-dimensional portrayal of the Mickey Mouse character of the comics, able to colonize and in some way alter the patient's world of introjective and projective identifications, recalls the concept of Bion's (1957) *bizarre object*. The comic, as well as the animated cartoon of Mickey Mouse, had been infused, so to speak, in the patient's psychotic experience with some infantile qualities of his own personality and projected outward by Miguel.

The concomitant action of uncontrollable urination during the analytic session appeared to be a dissociative attack of a somatic kind on the therapeutic alliance. It was as if the patient had intuited my initial resistance to becoming what he was unconsciously forcing me to be: namely, Mickey Mouse. Miguel could not give a name to any of his emotions or find a verbalizable meaning for his internal states, but, at the same time, he seemed to resist the analytic process that would have led him to some form of new awareness, a form that was terrifying for him. He used language as action—as demonstrated in his verbal expression aimed at me "You make me laugh, Mickey Mouse"—and the action of urinating in my office as language. He thereby communicated, through bodily transference, the aggression originally aimed in a dissociated way toward his mother.

When not openly communicated by the patient, access to a primal image— understood as "a picture of the patient in some infantile relationship to the psychiatrist, or, at any rate, to somebody" (Berne, 1977a [1955], p. 91)—is a function of the therapist's intuition. As the work with Miguel demonstrates, because the therapist's intuition is relative to aspects of the transference by the patient, the therapist often finds himself or herself handling (in supervision as well) a series of visual and polysensory experiences that are particularly disturbing and that risk conflicting notably with countertransference experiences that are similarly archaic (subsymbolic) relative to their own primary pre-object and object relationships. For these reasons, Berne advised that "there is nothing disreputable about intuition, since its most mystifying manifestations are based on infantile experiences, and for that reason are to be treated with respect, but also with caution" (p. 96).

In summary, the methodological assumption behind the therapist's active participation in the patient's *primal imaging* is that by the therapist retaining his or her clinical intuition and thoughts about bodily images—the "thinking sphincter," as Berne (1975b [1972], p. 357) described it—as an integral part of his or her bodily-emotional countertransference, and, as such, a protocol (i.e., subsymbolic) instrument, the therapist can remain actively involved in the analysis of bodily transactions that emerge in the here and now of the analytic relationship.

Listening

In transactional analysis in general, as in other forms of psychotherapy that are mainly based on spoken language, the use of words is central to the progression of the therapy. However, rather than the so-called "talking cure" that some therapies achieve, in the end, TA is, above all, a "listening cure."

Berne (1975b [1972], pp. 359–364) dedicated an entire chapter to "how to listen." He sought to offer, in his usual way, as exhaustive a list as possible of auditory cues through which to access a patient's script. I do not aim to offer here a critical revision of Berne's thinking in this regard but rather to recover the basic methodological position concerning active listening by the therapist during the analytic process. In particular, Berne commented that "his Adult [the analyst] listens to the content of what the patient says, while his Child-Professor listens to the way he [the patient] says it" (p. 361).

This *acoustic attunement*, which Berne saw as the fundamental requirement for a good listener, is indispensable in work with patients in active psychosis. For them, the main (if not the only) way in acute psychotic states of listening to the other, including the therapist, is with their Child.

In clinical situations, the intonation of the therapist's voice, its volume and rhythm, the timing of his or her verbal transactions, even (and sometimes especially) in the absence of visual exchanges, are among the sounds to which the psychotic patient is particularly attentive during therapy. One might say that the patient's internal acoustic disposition, coming from the most nuclear aspects of his or her Child, once again invites the therapist into a relationship similar to that lived by the original couple of primary caregiver (mother and/or father and/or significant others) and newborn. In this regard, Sabbadini (2014) wrote about how

> another aspect of mirroring, in parallel to the visual one described by Winnicott (1967), concerns the reflection of the child's voice, sounds, and noises—a process I propose here to call "echoing." ... For echoing to take place, the empathic and containing voice of [his] carers is an indispensable sounding-board, or resonance box, to the child's voice.
>
> (p. 126)

These considerations are themselves echoed in a number of works by earlier authors such as Cremerius (1969) and Anzieu (1989), for whom the earliest and most significant relational experiences between primary caregivers and newborn have a highly auditory quality: "The sound space is the first psychical space" (Anzieu, 1989, p. 170).

My first home visits to Anisha, whom I described earlier, went precisely in the opposite direction to that anticipated by Berne in his art of listening. Not only did she appear to be "blind" to the reality of her isolation and existential suffering, but I too had become partially "deaf" to the appeal from her internal world. This occurred to the point where my acoustic *misattunement* had become much more than a rejection of her spoken truth and had been perceived by her as a genuine threat to her integrity. The result, as described earlier, was a sudden breaking off of that initial, albeit minimal and fragile, relational harmony, an unforeseen, although probably feared, interruption in our communication. This was mainly caused by the fact that, although I was interested with my Adult in the content of what Anisha was trying to say, she was instead focused on the way I was listening and responding to her Child.

However, when the therapist is a good listener in the relationship with a schizophrenic patient, he or she quickly allows his or her Adult, listening to suggestions coming from his or her Child, to talk in the way an adult would with a real child. In these situations, therapists tend to favor a tone of voice that is less harsh and more gentle or lower pitched; the rhythm of their speech slows so they can pay attention to a sign or a grimace from the patient; and they use more filler words—such as "uh," "ah," "um," and "wow"—than usual to allow the conversation to unfold slowly. This reinforces an almost tacit understanding, surprise (also playfulness), exhortation, or genuine attention to what the patient is saying and goes on to say, sometimes even when the therapist remains completely silent. This particular aspect of auditory attunement constitutes a sort of *acoustic holding* that allows the patient not only to say words but also produce simple sounds—in some cases even grotesque or terrifying verses (metallic, animal noises, etc.), to stop and listen to them, even to enjoy them, and ultimately to recognize them as his or her own.

For example, Nathan, a fine arts student recently turned 20, the son of Somali parents but born and raised in the borough of Southwark in London, had a strange way of sighing during our sessions. In fact, these were like suppressed sighs, almost involuntary, which seemed like quick sucks of air, almost silent and always accompanied by a slight shudder in his chest. These seemed like quick moments of alarm, and right from the start I attributed to them an emotional significance of fear. A particularly interesting aspect of them was their unpredictability during the course of a session, which led to an uncomfortable state of anticipation waiting for those sighs and, in certain situations, even caused me to jump suddenly and almost imperceptibly in a similar way. At first I made a deliberate decision to ignore this phenomenon precisely to avoid this state of continual and irritating semialertness until, after a time, Nathan revealed to me that he was particularly worried about the way in which I handled my half-liter bottle of fizzy water, which I regularly brought with me, during the sessions.

(P = Patient, T = Therapist)

T: "What is it that worries you about this bottle?"
P: "It's because you close the cap very tightly when you close it."
T: "Yes ... I do that so that the air doesn't escape."

    Long pause. At that point I remarked that I had noticed that he sighed during the sessions, and I wondered whether he was worried or even frightened about something. He looked at me in fear and said, "How do you know?"

T: "Know what?" I said dubiously.
P: "How can you read my thoughts?"

After another pause, using the concrete object of the bottle as a metaphor (see the section on "Illustration" in Chapter 8) to talk about Nathan's perception of me (and, in a broader sense, of the therapy), I tried to ask him whether he was convinced that I could read his thoughts and whether he believed I could capture them inside the bottle, as I did with the air. With a similar level of concern, he not only agreed with my hypothesis but also declared that the way in which I brought the bottle close to my mouth, very slowly unscrewing the cap, between sips, showed how I inhaled his "last thoughts" trapped in the air of the bottle and swallowed those thoughts, which were already "diluted." I was dumbfounded by Nathan's anguished revelations, and I gathered them together as a brilliant explanation of what is meant in the psychoanalytic literature by projective and introjective identification, which, in Nathan's case, I thought to be underlying his psychotic experiences of the reading and stealing of his thoughts.

As the analysis progressed, Nathan even managed to remember that when he was a child, he often saw his father, who was a bricklayer at the time, come home from work really upset (perhaps already drunk) and start drinking poor-quality wine during dinner until he was drunk. These scenes were imbued with indescribable anguish because, at the slightest sign of complaint from Nathan's mother, a row would break out between the two of them, so violent that it would culminate in acts of physical aggression by his father toward his mother. Nathan had further associated his father's compulsive drinking with his father's anger about how his family was descending into near poverty and with the figurative "murder" of any thought that would be contrary to what his father would have felt at that time about work, family, and life in general.

This example shows how the patient's primal protocol still "re-sounds" in the analytic relationship as a kind of reverberant leitmotif with the potential to develop, with help from the sensory and emotional holding enabled by the therapy, into something more articulate. When on this wavelength, the therapist can enact—and often does so without full awareness—a protocol countertransference with anaclitic values, whether that be to foster the patient's need to be heard by the therapist in his or her role as a new Other or to stimulate the patient to listen to himself or herself in that moment. The aim is to enable the patient, over time, to focus on the way he or she relates to the sounds, even the almost imperceptible ones, emanating from his or her own body (as in Nathan's case), on the emotions that arise from them, and on the thoughts associated with them. This way of proceeding through the senses makes it possible for therapists to encourage in schizophrenic individuals a new, unprecedented way of systematically caring for themselves until they develop an increasingly coherent narrative of their own multiple experiences of life.

There is no shortage of repeated and sometimes exhaustingly long silences in work with psychotic patients. These can powerfully permeate the therapy room, constituting one of the biggest challenges the analyst faces as he or she cautiously, as well as courageously on a methodological level, attempts to achieve an analytic understanding of their transactional significance. I generally favor a theoretical shift away from the classical psychoanalytic concept of considering silence—similar to what initially occurred with transference and countertransference—unilaterally as a kind of resistance to the work of analysis based on *Freie Einfälle* (free association) as originally propounded by Freud (1953 [1900]). I instead consider it to be a transactional phenomenon that exists only within a relational exchange. In this way, silence, or at least the kind experienced in work with psychotic patients, can be understood more often than not as a duplex transaction but of a kind that is more specific than what Berne suggested, that is, a duplex transaction in which both the social level and the psychological level coincide. From this results the powerful confusional charge of silent transactions in work with schizophrenic individuals, which may explain why these transactions seem particularly close to dreamlike material.

With this in mind, it is reasonable to hypothesize a new rule of transactional communication: when the social message and the psychological message of a duplex transaction coincide, communication can only continue within an interbodily relationship. This is closer to the concept of a "relational field" or of a dreamlike and protomental dimension of thought. Access to psychological (and therefore social) content conveyed through the schizophrenic patient's silent transactions is, again, a task for analysts' Little Professor and thereby for their primal images and judgments (Berne, 1977a [1955], Chapter 4). This includes their "thinking sphincter" (Berne, 1975b [1972], p. 357), their intuition, and their protocol, from which stem their talent and their cursed incompetence in profound analytic work with these patients.

To put it methodologically, the main task of the therapist in this area of *acoustic exploration* is to clarify with the patient the reason for the latter's silence at that moment and to gather together all the signals emanating from the therapist's own body through his or her other senses, primal images, coenesthetic experiences, and emotional impressions aroused by the silence in that phase of the therapy.

The following clinical case vignette concerns part of a short transactional analysis treatment with Veronique, a patient just over 20 years old, originally from the Ivory Coast, clearly fragmented, and treated in the hospital within a multidisciplinary setting for several months. For organizational reasons, the therapy she received was of limited duration (i.e., the length of her hospitalization) and consisted of almost daily sessions. It included the active contribution of psychotropic medications aimed at containing the more serious episodes of psychotic anguish and dealing with her insomnia, which had already lasted around three weeks and left the patient prey to persecutory experiences involving the nurses and doctors on the ward.

One summer morning I was in my office alone, focused on completing a patient report, when Veronique stormed into the room and slammed the door behind her, holding it shut with one hand firmly holding the handle. Outside, the nurse could be heard, having rushed to the scene, pleading with Veronique to allow her in. The patient was still in her pajamas. On her loose top a large, coffee-colored ring could clearly be seen on her chest, showing the point of a nipple in relief. She remained silent with her face showed signs of exhaustion after yet another sleepless night. She looked at me, her eyes filling with tears as she shouts at me in a rage, "Monster, that's what you are, a monster!" It was only at that point that she loosened her grip on the door handle, thus allowing the nurse to enter the room. Meanwhile, Veronique carefully sat down on the chair in front of the desk. She continued to stare at me but with an expression that had suddenly become contrite. She continued to hurl insults at me, even maintaining that the stain on her pajamas had to do with my "dirty semen," repeating in a calm but accusatory tone of voice, "You went away, you ugly shitface, see how you left me dirty" while continuing to point at the stain on her top.

This illustrates one of the difficulties posed by schizophrenic psychosis, which is the eroticization of the relationship. I made a mental note that this tantrum was probably linked to my unexpected absence from work for about a week following an intensive period of daily meetings during which Veronique had talked several times, sometimes quite explicitly, about sexual fantasies to do with another patient. Her accusations now centered on her perception, very vivid in her mind, of having been physically "violated" by me. I interpreted this, again in my head, as a defense against the strong threat stemming from the reawakening of her female sexuality and, at the same time, her progressive awareness, arising from our discourse, of her solitude and unshakable fear of men and other people in general. Simultaneously, I had the feeling that the open attack on me, in the episode described here, was a different attempt, born of desperation as much as anything else, to maintain close contact with me. Veronique had shown a strong inclination to create a "special" relationship with me to the point of fantasizing a love affair between us that had seemed to her increasingly real because of our frequent conversations and meetings, as much as several times a day during her stay in the hospital. With me suddenly gone for a week, she had felt "violated," that is to say, violated in the purity and virginity of her confessions and her most intimate fantasies about me. Ultimately, she felt "soiled," rejected and despised due to my unexpected absence.

As the sessions progressed, I realized increasingly, with a certain mingled relief, that what Veronique wanted was also and more profoundly this: that I was clearer with her, less "soiled," that is, less turbid and enigmatic with my intellectual interpretations and more open to her most intimate fantasies. I ended up reading in her a desperate need not only to feel listened to but also comforted as she suddenly perceived herself to be alone and fragile. She wanted ultimately to be accepted and loved as a grown woman rather than just as a patient.

This episode with Veronique shows the evocative power of images attributed to certain obscene words spoken by the patient, what Ferenczi called "obscene verbal images."

> An obscene word has a peculiar power of compelling the hearer to imagine the object it denotes, the sexual organ or function, in *substantial actuality*. ... These words as such possess the capacity of compelling the hearer to revive memory pictures in a regressive and hallucinatory manner. ... The obscene verbal images retain as does all repressed material the characters of a more primitive type of imagination.
>
> (Ferenczi as cited by Berne, 1977a [1955], pp. 70–71)

In Veronique's case, the obscene words she expressed verbally evoked in me intrusive and, more subtly, olfactory sexual images (particularly sweat and sperm), to the point where they provoked a kind of disgust mixed with a feeling of great embarrassment. This confirms the crossmodal (i.e., belonging to more than one sensory modality) nature of the act of perception—which is mainly polysensory and synesthetic—by the Child and hence by the psychophysiological activity of the bodily ego.

Schizophrenic patients are also greater listeners to voices than other people, which further explains the reason for some of the silences in therapy. As with other sensory experiences, there exists a huge literature that describes auditory experiences in schizophrenic psychoses, distinguishing them into the categories of hallucinations, pseudohallucinations, hallucinosis, and illusions. This literature is the subject of descriptive psychopathology and phenomenological psychopathology. The reader, and even more the psychotherapist, is therefore encouraged to consult the existing literature on the phenomenology of schizophrenic psychosis.

In the structural analysis of psychoses originally proposed by Berne, visual and auditory hallucinations (the latter the most common encountered in clinical practice) are mainly attributed to contaminations in the structure of the primal order and usually come from the Parent (P_2) and/or the Child (C_2) ego states. The theory proposed here (see Chapter 3) shifts the area of interest with regard to these hallucinatory experiences (as is the case with delusions) onto the self (Mellacqua, 2014) and therefore onto internal experiences and transactional processes of the Child. This is where a person's *feeling of reality* resides, including the reality of one's own sensory and bodily self, what one is insofar as one "feels" oneself to be. Bollas (2015) argued similarly when he wrote, "Indeed, the voices originate from distinct parts of the child self" (p. 105). More than this, the schizophrenic's repeated experiences of hearing voices, similar to what happens with sensory experiences linked to other sense organs, are subject to the rules of splitting, projection, and introjection. As "repudiated portion[s] of the self" (pp. 105–106), these voices can inhabit physical objects in the external world and therefore be attributed to apparently inanimate objects (e.g., a house, a mobile phone, etc.), to natural features (e.g., a river, a plant, etc.), and so on. It is the nature of self-referentiality—the fact of being repeatedly referred back to the psychotic individual—that makes the hallucinations (not just auditory ones) tend to be ego-syntonic, that is, experiences the patient deceptively believes can be perceived in the physical reality surrounding his or her own ego. Deconstructing this illusory quality of hallucinations means to undermine, as Bollas (2015) wrote, the illusory nature of having a univocal ego. Thus, analytic work on hallucinatory experiences (often accompanied by more or less structured delusions) is one of the most challenging tasks—although, on a human level, also one of the most compelling—that the therapist experiences with schizophrenic patients.

For example, Marco, about 45 years old and affected by a chronic form of hebephrenic schizophrenia, was often observed sitting alone with his legs crossed in a corner of the ward. On closer inspection, I could see that he was intent on "writing" (sans pen) with his right index finger at the level of his left knee. This was one of the ways in which he appeared absorbed in a kind of inner bubble composing who knows what phrase or thought. One day the curiosity to know more about this somewhat bizarre activity of "invisible writing" got the better of me, and, approaching him carefully, I attempted to engage him in conversation.

(P = Patient, T = Therapist)

T: "Hi Marco."

P: "Hi"

T: "I can see you're concentrating, can I ask what you're doing?"

P: "Can't you see? I'm writing." He continued undisturbed to make actual writing movements with his finger.

I stood there in silence for almost a minute trying to spot a word in the movements Marco was making but that were indecipherable to me. At a certain point, I said, "Can I ask what you're writing?"

After a pause, he whispered to me, "Prudenza, Pazienza, Speranza" [i. e., Caution, Patience, Hope].

T: "Ah … what's that? What did you say?"

P: "Detto. Matto. Morto." [Said. Mad. Dead.]

I was a bit puzzled and then added, "Do you like rhymes?"

P: "Yes."

T: "I'm wondering though, Marco, that if you are writing Prudenza, Pazienza, Speranza [Caution, Patience, Hope] whether this means something to you."

Silence.

T: "Are you perhaps telling yourself that you have to be cautious, patient, and that you have to have hope? Or is it something you're also advising others to have … do you understand what I mean?"

P: "Yes, it's for me; caution, patience, hope." At that point he actually interrupted his invisible writing and added, "It helps me. Detto. Matto. Morto" [Said. Mad. Dead].

T: "Is that why you write it like that? In that way with your finger, because it's only for you?"

P: "If I can't talk, then I'll write." He lifts his head and looks at me almost fearfully, then looks away and returns to his writing, adding: "See? I write. I write about me."

It took several further meetings like this one for Marco to explain what he was actually doing when he took himself away to "write." Over the years, it was the only way he had found to deal with the "voices in his head," which repeatedly told him that he was a "bastard" and insistently ordered him to "shut up." "Shut up, you bastard," they said to him, "Shut up!" So one day he had told himself that if he was not able to talk, he could surely write, and so no one would know he had found a way of tricking the voices with a "special" tool, his finger, using "invisible" ink and even writing something misleading and vague compared with what the voices were saying. Thus he wrote, "Prudenza, Pazienza, Speranza" [Caution, Patience, Hope].

As our sessions progressed during his stay on the ward, Marco went on to clarify that there was more than one voice in his head, although he was unable to quantify the exact number. The words he had chosen to write

145

repeatedly on his body had instead become for him a means of "coping with the negativity of the voices," even a way of making his thoughts invisible, of hiding himself. He became increasingly distressed as he managed to talk to me about his "special writings," as he once called them. He was frightened that the voices might order him to do something bad, although this never came to pass. In fact, he was able, guided by simple questions aimed at investigating the presumed origin of these voices, to remember certain traumatic episodes from his primary school years. At that time he had been the victim of verbal and even physical abuse—what we would now call bullying—by other pupils at school. I also knew that Marco was the son of a teenage mother and had never known his father, who was apparently an Algerian immigrant. The negative voices in his head were, therefore, primarily linked to his personal history and to successive traumatic experiences during his first years at school. These had reinforced and amplified his ontological fragility and ultimately had become split parts of his own nuclear self. They were then defensively projected out by the Child ego state but were still able to return to it repeatedly and intrusively in the form of denigratory and domineering voices.

As these clinical excerpts show, the main task of the transactional analyst in these circumstances goes beyond empathic understanding of the patient's auditory experiences. The aim, instead, is to sharpen the patient's ability to listen more reflectively to these acoustic, although disturbing, experiences, which, like all primal images, have a strong impact at a bodily-emotional level. The objective guiding this process of colistening between therapist and patient is, once again, an analytic one. It is to investigate, with the patient's active contribution in the here and now, the number of voices (whether one or more), the content (what they say or whether they are indistinct voices similar to murmuring or noise), the possible identity or origin of the voice(s) in structural terms (whether a memory of someone or something from the subject's past), their spatial location and proximity (whether outside or inside the head, whether far away or near), the context in which they occur (whether certain events or situations trigger them), the type of relationship with the self (whether they are benevolent or malevolent), and the bodily-emotional resonance of the voices (whether they induce anguish, terror, behavioral aggression or, in contrast, comfort, relief, calm).

The result of this approach is a progressive weakening of the sense that the voice(s) are alien to the self and guidance of the patient toward increasing awareness, in line with Berne's position, of the intrinsic plurality of the ego, which is seen—also through the experience of auditory hallucinations—in a multiplicity of mental states.

Tasting and smelling

Taste and smell are dealt with together here both because, on a biological level, one is usually functionally connected with the other, and because in clinical conditions (with some exceptions), unpleasant olfactory experiences are often reported by patients alongside taste reactions and/or other hallucinations.

What follows is a brief description of the case of a 30-year-old patient, Sonia, already known to the local psychiatric services for about six months for a probable onset of paranoid schizophrenia. She had been sent to me for psychotherapeutic support while in weekly day-hospital care under the supervision of a psychodynamically oriented clinical psychologist.

Sonia's persecutory symptoms had started a few months previously and were concentrated on the negative interference in her life of a male colleague. He had apparently made repeated allusions at work, and in the presence of other colleagues, about a presumed homosexual relationship of the patient. At our first therapy session, Sonia reported feeling persecuted almost daily by this colleague but said she was single and denied any form of romantic relationship with other women. It was not clear if she was having any hallucinatory experiences.

Subsequent sessions focused on taking a more detailed history and building a therapeutic relationship. My aim to follow her for weekly therapy for at least a year was interrupted, however, for the first time in only the sixth session.

(P = Patient, T = Therapist)

P: "You stink of alcohol like my father. You disgust me as a therapist and as a man. Ugh!"

T: [Silence and then in a resentful tone] "I'd like you to know that I don't drink wine before a therapy session. What makes you think that I am an alcoholic?"

P: "Look here … you just said it … how disgusting! … I'm not going to talk to you any more."

That session became the subject of work with my clinical supervisor, who asked me first to recount my own and the patient's verbal exchange (as just described) and second to say something about my impressions, particularly on an emotional and bodily level, in response to the patient's "accusations" against me. After that he asked me why I had chosen to bring this case to supervision. This is an excerpt of that supervision.

(S = Supervisor, T = Therapist)

S: "Give me your impressions of the patient's sensory experiences."

T: "I think that in this session the patient reported a clear olfactory sensation that had all the hallmarks of being a hallucinatory phenomenon."

S: "Um … that doesn't tell me anything about the patient's internal world or about the quality of her relationships with her primary figures"… [silence].

T: "Well, a hallucination is a perception without object …" [in a slightly irritated tone]

S: "It is nevertheless a perception by the subject …"

T: "Actually, I analytically linked her olfactory experience to her personal history."

S: "How?"

T: "The patient had an alcoholic father who died young, I believe around the age of 26, when she was about 10 years old, in a road accident. I got this information in previous sessions."

S: "Um … good … moreover the patient herself has told you that you remind her of her father."

T: "Yes, that's true … I thought that the patient's sensory perception, which is associated with the distinctive smell of wine, made her think of her father. … She screamed at me she was so disgusted … It was her negative transference onto me…"

S: "Um … this shows you are jumping to intellectual conclusions already, although they are probably valid."

T: "I don't understand."

S: "The point is not to understand first … but what did you feel when she told you that you stank like her father?"

T: "That she was attacking me unjustly. I perceived hatred and disgust toward me … and obviously toward her father."

S: "If you had been able to do anything, what would you have done?"

T: "Do?"

S: "Yes, do. What would you have done with her if you had been able to?"
[After a moment's reflection]

T: "Well, I would have refuted her. I felt invaded by those accusations … I thought she was paranoid toward me too."

S: "Which is what others do with her … they stay well away from her …"

T: "Yes, it's exactly like that …"

S: "And what happened then?"

T: "She suddenly broke off the session and she left"… [silence]

S: "Um … there's a part missing, don't you think?

T: "Um … I don't know…"

S: "How on earth you stank of alcohol …"

T: "Hey, here we go again … perceptions without object … I think she was hallucinating … in her mind I stank of wine like her father."

S: "I'd like to point out to you that the patient spoke of alcohol … not wine …"

My supervisor's reflection on that metonymy between the terms "alcohol" (used by the patient) and "wine" (used by me based on information from her personal history) left me confused for a moment and also annoyed.

Although the patient cancelled the following two sessions, I continued to work with her for around another six months before she asked to be transferred to a female therapist. During the work with her, however, I was able to confirm my supervisor's intuitions. Her father's alcoholism was much more serious than I had thought. When Sonia was still a little girl, her father was a young man whose dependence on drugs and alcohol had even led him to drink the ethyl alcohol liquids inside alcohol-based deodorants and aftershaves. His death at a relatively young age, a similar age to my own at the time, made negative transference by the patient toward me more likely (at the time I was a still a junior therapist in training). Despite all of this, I would never have imagined that using an aftershave, as opposed to my normal balsam for sensitive skin, would have been able to change the course of the analytic therapy with this patient.

I still remember vividly in a subsequent session with Sonia being struck by an internal vision in which I saw her at preschool age in her father's arms trying to get away from being kissed by him. Perhaps this was why she could not stand the strong and nauseating smell of alcohol. Once again, this type of vision had the characteristics of a primal image, that is, "a picture of the patient in some infantile relationship to the psychiatrist, or, at any rate, to somebody" (Berne, 1977a [1955], p. 91). This was a kind of "olfactory relationship" (Lemma, 2015, p. 20) reenacted through bodily transference—like other extra-analytic relationships that Sonia talked about in sessions—that provided valuable information on the nature of her object (and, if you like, also preobject) relationship with her paternal figure. This represented her attraction to male figures (including the therapist) and, at the same time, her repulsion of these relationships, which she perceived as intoxicating, potentially seductive, and intrusive.

Later on in the work with Sonia, welcoming in the analytic setting the patient's subjective experience of the Other (P_1) based on smell, I had, in fact, substituted my usual balsam aftershave with an alcohol-based one for a period of about 10 days. This allowed the patient's sense organ—now as well as in her infancy and early adolescence—to be placed at the service of her ego in order to develop her awareness of her own bodily identity, of almost ineffable emotions in relation to actual significant others, and even of her sexuality.

Finally, this case formally introduced me, and through the recommendation of my then-supervisor, to the work of the psychoanalyst Didier Anzieu (1989, 1990 [1987]) and his ideas of *skin-ego* and *psychic envelope*. In time I also discovered and further appreciated the value of some of Berne's (1977a [1955], 1975b [1972], pp. 291–294) more powerful and pioneering observations on primal images and, in particular, on smell, and their social importance: "Smell imagery is characteristic of primal images. So is taste, or at any rate, internal sensations" (Berne, 1977a [1955], p. 77).

References

Anzieu, D. (1989). *The skin ego: A psychoanalytic approach to the self*. New Haven, CT: Yale University Press.

Anzieu, D. (1990). *Psychic envelope*. London: Karnac Books. (Original work published 1987)

Benedetti, G. (1997). *La psicoterapia come sfida esistenziale* [Psychotherapy as existential challenge]. Milan: Cortina. (Original work published 1992)

Berne, E. (1975a). *Transactional analysis in psychotherapy: A systematic individual and social psychiatry*. London: Souvenir Press. (Original work published 1961)

Berne, E. (1975b). *What do you say after you say hello? The psychology of human destiny*. London: Corgi. (Original work published 1972)

Berne, E. (1977a). Primal images and primal judgment. In E. Berne, P. McCormick (Ed.) *Intuition and ego states: The origins of transactional analysis* (pp. 67–97). San Francisco, CA: TA Press. (Original work published 1955)

Berne, E. (1977b). *Principles of group treatment*. New York, NY: Grove Press. (Original work published 1966)

Bick, E. (1968). The experience of the skin in early object relations. *International Journal of Psychoanalysis*, 29, 484–486.

Bick, E. (2002). Further considerations on the function of the skin in early object relations. In A. Briggs (Ed.), *Surviving space: Papers on infant observation* (pp. 60–71). London: Karnac Books. (Original work published 1986)

Bion, W. R. (1957). Differentiation of the psychotic from the non-psychotic. *International Journal of Psychoanalysis*, 38, 206–275.

Bion, W. R. (1961). *Experiences in groups and other papers*. New York, NY: Basic Books.

Bion, W. R. (1984). *Second thoughts: Selected papers on psycho-analysis*. London: Karnac Books. (Original work published 1967)

Bloom, K. (2006). *The embodied self: Movement and psychoanalysis*. London: Karnac Books.

Bollas, C. (2015). *When the sun bursts: The enigma of schizophrenia*. New Haven, CT: Yale University Press.

Bucci, W. (1997). *Psychoanalysis and cognitive science: A multiple code theory*. New York, NY: Guilford.

Bucci, W. (2008). The role of bodily experience in emotional organisation. In F. S. Anderson (Ed.), *Bodies in treatment: The unspoken dimension* (pp. 51–76). New York, NY: The Analytic Press.

Bucci, W. (2011). The role of embodied communication in therapeutic change. In W. Tschachen & C. Bergoni (Eds.), *The implications of embodiment: Cognition and communication* (pp. 209–229). Charlottesville, VA: Imprint-Academic.

Cornell, W. F. (2015). *Somatic experience in psychoanalysis and psychotherapy: In the expressive language of the living*. London: Routledge.

Cremerius, J. (1969). Schweigen als problem der psychoanalytischen technik [Silence as a problem of psychoanalytic technology]. *Jahrbuck der Psychoanalyse*, 6, 69–103.

Freud, S. (1953). The interpretation of dreams. In J. Strachey (Ed. & Trans.), *The standard edition of the complete psychological works of Sigmund Freud* (Vol. 4, pp. 1–338; Vol. 5, pp. 339–630). London: Hogarth Press. (Original work published 1900)

Freud, S. (1958a). Formulations on the two principles of mental functioning. In J. Strachey (Ed. & Trans.), *The standard edition of the complete psychological works of Sigmund Freud* (Vol. 12, pp. 218–226). London: Hogarth Press. (Original work published 1911)

Freud, S. (1958b). Three essays on the theory of sexuality. In J. Strachey (Ed. & Trans.), *The standard edition of the complete psychological works of Sigmund Freud* (Vol. 7, pp. 123–245). London: Hogarth Press. (Original work published 1905)

Garfield, D. A. S. (2009). *Unbearable affect: A guide to the psychotherapy of psychosis.* London: Karnac Books. (Original work published 2005)

Lemma, A. (2015). *Minding the body: The body in psychoanalysis and beyond.* London: Routledge.

Lombardi, R., & Pola, M. (2010). The body, adolescence, and psychosis. *The International Journal of Psychoanalysis, 91,* 1419–1444.

McDougall, J. (1989). *Theaters of the body: A psychoanalytic approach to psychosomatic illness.* New York, NY: Norton.

McDougall, J. (1995). *The many faces of Eros: A psychoanalytic exploration of human sexuality.* New York, NY: Norton.

Mellacqua, Z. (2014). Beyond symbiosis: The role of primal exclusions in schizophrenia psychosis. *Transactional Analysis Journal, 44,* 8–10.

Merleau-Ponty, M. (1986). *The phenomenology of perception* (C. Smith, Trans.). London: Routledge and Kegan Paul. (Original work published 1945)

Resnik, S. (2001). *Persona e psicosi* [Person and psychosis]. Turin: Einaudi. (Original work published 1972)

Resnik, S. (2002). *L'esperienza psicotica* [The psychotic experience]. Turin: Bollati Boringheri. (Original work published 1986)

Resnik, S. (2005). *Glacial times: A journey through the world of madness.* New York, NY: Routledge.

Resnik, S. (2007). *Il teatro del sogno* [The theater of the dream]. Turin, Italy: Bollati Boringheri. (Original work published 1982)

Sabbadini, A. (2014). *Boundaries and bridges: Perspectives on time and space in psychoanalysis.* London: Karnac Books.

Sarte, J. P. (1992). *Being and nothingness: A phenomenological essay on ontology* (H. E. Barnes, Trans.). New York, NY: Washington Square Press. (Original work published 1943)

Winnicott, W. D. (1971). *Playing and reality.* London: Tavistock.

Woollams, S., & Brown, M. (1978). *Transactional analysis.* Dexter, MI: Huron Valley Institute.

7

COUNTERTRANSFERENCE IN THE FACE OF PSYCHOSIS

The discussion of countertransference here begins with the principle that the analyst's countertransference, inasmuch as it is the result of unconscious communication arising from the intimate relationship within the analysis, is inevitably affected by the informative influence and interference provided by the patient's transference. It is always, to use Resnik's (2007 [1982]) words, a double perspective or double transference, a bipersonal context, therefore a *joint responsibility* (p. 57). Consequently, this section will expand on the therapeutic role of countertransference for both the patient and the analyst, explaining, in particular, its use in work with individuals affected by schizophrenia and, more generally, by a psychotic level of self-disturbance.

Bodily-emotional coinduction

Within the analytic relationship, the paranoid patient projects both idealized aspects and persecutory elements of his or her nonintegrated internal object world directly onto the therapist, who then experiences episodes of indescribable anguish, unusual muscular tensions, and even blocks in the body. In both idealized and persecutory situations, countertransference actions or inactions represent a difficult and desperate attempt to escape from this disturbing position in which the therapist sees a threat to the integration of his or her own self and therefore to the sense of personal identity that preceded the development of a professional identity.

Strange as it may seem, the outcome of countertransference, in terms of emotional experiences, is always the polar opposite of what is experienced by the paranoid patient during projective transference. In a broader sense, this once again demonstrates the informative capacity of countertransference experienced by the therapist about the patient's experiences (Racker, 1982 [1968]). So, for example, if the patient is strongly convinced of his or her own beliefs, the analyst is assailed by doubt about having made an irredeemable mistake in his or her own conjectures and intentions; if the analyst feels particularly in control of his or her own actions, the patient feels lost and at the mercy of the analyst; if the analyst experiences aggression, the patient feels threatened; and so on.

As mentioned earlier (see section "Projective counteridentification" in Chapter 4), projective counteridentification can also lead to a progressive affective estrangement by the therapist due to a counterdissociation and the use of intellectual interpretations too early in the therapeutic process. The result of this kind of behavior on the part of the therapist is often a breakdown in the therapeutic alliance and even premature termination of the therapy.

The therapeutic use of projective counteridentification stems from recognizing that this countertransference process is primarily a defense used by the therapist to resolve the anguish of splitting induced in him or her by the analytic relationship, just as the psychotic patient does during projective identification. Consequently, as a defense, projective counteridentification allows the therapist to maintain internal equilibrium but at the cost of procedural near paralysis. The analyst's task is then to interrupt the counter-identification in favor of *containing* emotional experiences of hatred (or, conversely, self-satisfaction) and, at the same time, of anguish channeled by the paranoid patient.

Containment should not be viewed as the therapist passively receiving the patient's projections. Instead, it is a relational system through which the therapist is charged with induced emotions providing—like a kind of thermal conductor—on the one hand, the human warmth the patient needs in order to (re)include the primarily excluded Parent in the analytic relationship and, on the other, to receive a signal—like a thermal sensor would give—about the intensity of the emotional experiences projected unconsciously onto the therapist.

However, relational containment in itself is not enough to regulate down the intensity of the patient's projective identification, which can lead to an emotional overheating with the further risk of triggering or intensifying the therapist's counteridentification. The analytic relationship can, therefore, continue and evolve in a transformative sense to the extent that the therapist uses his or her countertransference as a kind of variable internal resistance, that is, variably deflecting the emotions induced by the patient from one session to the next without extinguishing or silencing them. An effective psychotherapy, wrote Garfield (2009 [2005]), "even at the outset, requires making the unbearable more bearable" (p. 154). This therapeutic process, which I refer to as *emotional coinduction*, is consequently a function of the degree of relative "refractoriness" by the therapist of emotional experiences induced by the patient, against which the patient defends himself or herself and that he or she paradoxically needs in order to consciously reintegrate split parts of his or her own self. The main therapeutic goal of coinduction in psychosis is, therefore, to encourage the integration of fragments of the ego that act as multiple and distinct and thus not integrated personalities, the result of egoic splitting processes of a mainly vertical kind (see Chapter 3).

For example, Mr Blake (first described in Chapter 4) began one of his sessions by lingering once again on a series of often disconnected reflections about the origin of the universe and how the Big Bang theory was correct. I, on the other hand, felt particularly irritated because he stubbornly continued to wear his dark sunglasses.

(P = Patient, T = Therapist)

T: "I wonder when you intend to grace a session without wearing your glasses."

P: "Bang! And here we are ... eh, doctor?"

T: "What do you mean?"

P: "That things happen like that, with a bang!"

T: "Do you think that our meeting is also the result of a Bang?"

P: "Zephyrus ... you're not a planet though."

T: "Certainly not. I like the Greek pronunciation."

P: "You are the wind, the wind everywhere ... Zephyrus ...Virus."

T: "Virus? What does 'virus' have to do with it?"Mr Blake's speech was particularly cryptic in that session, but I gradually became aware of a main theme around which his verbal offerings revolved. It concerned my presumed therapeutic and at the same time "infectious" abilities, which could endanger someone's health (including his own).

(P = Patient, T = Therapist)

P: "You stay on me."

T: "You mean that our sessions stay in your mind? What do you think about them between one session and the next?"

P: "On me. I said on me!"

T: "Um, you say on you ... you mean, if I understand right, it's like I am stuck to you ... like the wind, which attaches itself to skin, to clothes ... is it like that?"

P: "You can be here and there. Behind, in front, inside the ears."

T: "In the ears?"

P: "Yes, like thoughts in the ears, transparent." [A moment of silence. And then he starts again], "Can you really follow people anywhere?"

T: "Um ... are you saying that you feel followed by me?"

P: "I often see you in Brixton ... that is a fact."

T: "Well, as you know, I see lots of different planets (*lapsus linguae*) ... sorry, patients ... I see lots of different patients in their houses every day. I am often out and about, it's true."

P: Long pause. Then he adds, "It's amazing for a patient to see their own doctor around their own area and giving protection."

T: "You are saying that my presence can reassure you?" Another pause, and then I begin again saying: "But you also said 'virus' ... which means I can also be a danger to your health? A virus can cause an infection."

As this clinical excerpt demonstrates, the therapeutic goal of the transactional analyst in work with the paranoid person is primarily to contain the emotive experiences that are split off and induced in him or her by the patient, restoring them to the patient with gradually reduced intensity. This enables both a progressive reappropriation of emotive experiences that are unconsciously split and expelled by the ego and the operation and development of an affective regulation of these experiences.

(P = Patient, T = Therapist)

T: I went on, "The image that you describe of a doctor who's always moving around dispensing protection and reassurance in your area makes me feel as if I'm that doctor, do you understand? I mean, it makes me feel like a sort of superhero with superpowers. I'm everywhere, free, transparent as the wind, I can even influence other people's thoughts, and can therefore also get into your head. But then I also feel like a virus. Something dangerous. I'm invisible, but this time I can cause damage to people's health, to your health." Silence. While I'm waiting, I see him shake his head and then lean forward while remaining seated.

T: "At this point, Mr Blake, I wonder whether you also feel a bit like me. Namely, if ..."

P: "Don't play with me, doctor," he says while I see on a his face a grimace of a smile forming that suggests tacit assent immediately followed by sudden irritation.

T: For a moment I remain silent, disconcerted and a little afraid of his reaction. Then I calmly start again, telling him "I'm only trying to be myself, to listen to you and to tell you openly what I feel and think about what you are telling me in the session."

As Bollas (1987) clearly put it, "By cultivating a freely-aroused emotional sensibility, the analyst welcomes news from within himself that is reported through his own intuitions, feelings, passing images, phantasies. ... In order to find the patient we must look for him within ourselves" (p. 202).

When emotive conductance works, the patient feels listened to by someone and progressively produces experiences of psychotic anguish within the analytic relationship. This gradually reduces the possibility that these will come out in extra-analytic situations that could cause the person major problems in different areas of life. Within the analytic relationship, however, the patient becomes more open to transformative experiences through the recruitment of what Berne came to call the "Little Professor" (A_1), simultaneously integrating sensory, bodily-emotional, and thought experiences into ego states that over time become more coherent and mature.

Bodily-emotional deflection

Emotional deflection is particularly important when there is antagonistic transference onto the therapist, especially when there is a higher risk that the psychotic individual will turn to acts of self-harm or aggression toward others. Such situations are more frequent in institutional psychotherapy contexts such as psychiatric hospitals, forensic psychiatry wards, and rehabilitative psychiatry clinics. Through emotional deflection, the therapist rejects the antagonistic emotion (usually persistent malevolence and even physical threat) induced by the patient and silently deflects the induction.

During my time as a private clinical therapist in the London area of Elephant and Castle, I started seeing a couple of patients on Saturday morning. One of the inconvenient things about that time is the difficulty of finding a secretary. I decided, therefore, to take on the role of welcoming my Saturday patients and opening and shutting the office by myself. One day I became aware, in a way I perhaps never had before, of the risks involved in undertaking psychotherapy work with seriously ill patients in private alone in one's own office.

When I opened the door to John that Saturday, I was immediately aware that he seemed noticeably nervous and twitchy. I did not even have time to shut the door behind me before I saw him striding furiously toward my office. I tried to call his name, and he suddenly turned and pointed his finger threateningly at me while remaining at a distance of some meters and shouting at me, "Don't do it! Don't you dare!" before literally catapulting himself into my room and violently shutting the door.

Even today I find it hard to describe what went through my head in those minutes. They seemed very long as John stayed in my office. I was rigid with fear. An image came to mind that John might be in the grip of strong emotions and mounting psychomotor agitation, but, at the same time, I feared that he could come back and physically attack me. I sifted quickly in my head through the few bits of information I had about his history. I worked out that as far as I knew, John had never actually attacked anyone, and he did not use drugs or abuse alcohol. I also thought how stupid I was to see him on a Saturday morning alone. But in that situation, which was becoming increasingly uncomfortable for me, I did not manage to keep a cool head. I felt an indescribable tension. I had unconsciously picked up my telephone and was clumsily trying to scroll through my phone book or maybe call the secretary or even the police. I also thought about how long that would take. I thought that perhaps I should simply leave my office and ask for help outside. I had no idea what to do. The result was total paralysis. Several minutes passed until finally I attempted with shaking legs to approach the door to my office, which was now closed following the slam caused by the violent closure.

(P = Patient, T = Therapist)

T: "John? What's going on? Please John …" After a long silence, I tried to put my hand on the door handle, and John's response was another shout in which he literally ordered me to stay out, not to try to go in. After an interminable silence, I heard him say, "Liar! Liar!"

T: "John, I'm here to help you."

P: "Enough! I said enough!"

T: "John, let me come in, please."

P: "You want me to die! You want me to die in that shithouse … I'm dying like a mouse!"

T: "John, can I come in?" Another long silence. My legs felt very heavy. I was still frightened, but gradually I realized that John did not intend to leave my office. At least not straightaway.

I tried to tell him that I did not want either of us to get hurt, that I was afraid of his reactions, that a part of him hated this place (the therapy room) and was even ready to destroy it. I told him that a part of him probably hated me because I cast doubt on his convictions about the ultrasound and his neighbors (see also the section "Situating time in space" in Chapter 5 where the case of John is first presented). And perhaps, I thought, another part of him could not stand the fact that I was frightened of his behavior, as if my fear exacerbated his own and made him more disorganized. What I did not tell him then was that he was as frightened as I was and that the tremendous fear that he was inducing in me was the same fear of annihilation from which he was defending himself. When I finally managed to enter my office, with a resolve I was not actually feeling, I found John on his feet near the balcony with his head between his hands.

(P = Patient, T = Therapist)

T: "John, please."

P: "Beast!" he shouted. He turned suddenly and ran out, bumping my hip as he did so. "Beast!" he repeated. Then I heard noises from the street echoing round the room, a sign that John had left the entry door open. It was the last time I saw John. But that door left open made me hope for a long time that perhaps one day he would come back or, at least, that a little chink of awareness would sooner or later open in his mind, and perhaps he would ask again for help from someone.

The therapist's main aim in these scenarios tends to be to induce the patient to take back the projected emotion and recognize it as his or her own. This is easier said than done. John's case was proof of that for me. Bodily-emotional deflection, both silent and verbal, carries a greater risk of being perceived by the patient as either a lack of emotional responsiveness (or compliance) or an attack on his or her integrity. On this point, Semrad and Van Buskirk (1969) eloquently explained how the only thing that remains open to the vulnerable Ego is, at this point, suicide, murder or psychosis. Suicide and murder are the extreme expressions of emotion (especially rage) translated into action; psychosis is partial containment rationalised by emotion, the sacrifice of reality to preserve life.

(p. 23)

Emotional deflection should, consequently, be used with extreme caution, even with knowledge of the individual's psychobiography, the content of previous sessions, and the level of therapeutic alliance. The result of openly expressed emotional deflection can be an intensification of projective identification. This leads to projection onto the therapist not only of negative persecutory experiences (hate and psychophysical threat) but also idealized experiences of an omnipotent kind (reification) with deterioration in the paranoid psychosis leading to the development of experiences of psychotic influence, depersonalization, and derealization. These are extreme situations in which multidisciplinary work involving medical and nursing staff and the prescription of psychopharmacological medication aimed at reducing psychotic fragmentation and psychomotor agitation become almost indispensable. Only then can analytic work resume with a return to using containment as a way of tuning in again to the emotional experiences of the patient.

However, when emotional deflection is successful, it does allow the patient, as well as the therapist, to continue to think of reasonable options for their (i. e., of both the patient's and the therapist's) own psychophysical integrity as well as that of others, despite the presence of emotions intense enough to trigger potentially dangerous acts against themselves (i.e., the patient and the therapist) or others (usually significant others).

A more favorable outcome involves patients using more mature defenses, such as those that are protonarcissistic and object related. This allows them to gradually recognize the separateness of the therapist's ego with regard to emotional experiences that belong to their (i.e., the patient's) own ego. These are particularly fruitful developments in transactional analysis therapy with less acute schizophrenic patients who can increasingly tolerate the concomitant use of empathic transactions (Hargaden & Sills, 2002, Chapter 8) in the context of transference and countertransference dynamics brilliantly categorized by Kohut (1971) into mirroring transference/countertransference, idealizing transference/countertransference, and twinship transference/countertransference.

In light of this explanation, here is a clinical excerpt from the therapy with Alice, the young student who had manifested a growing existential anguish with vague persecutory experiences after moving to London to take up her university studies (see Chapter 5 under the section "Situating time in place or context").

(P = Patient, T = Therapist)

P: "I reached the conclusion that something is wrong inside me."

T: "What reasons do you have for thinking that about yourself?"

P: "Well, I have never passed even one exam, my family continues to pay for my studies and my rent, I can't make any social relationships, and I don't have a single friend, let alone a boy who I like who I could go out with every so often or go for a beer."

T: "In other words, Alice, you're telling me that you are a loser. And, in fact, that's what is really happening. Yes, you're a loser."

P: She looked at me, perplexed, and then stammered, "That's just what they tell me."

T: "Who tells you that? Apart from me today?" Silence.

T: "Do the voices tell you that?"

P: "What voices? No, that is ... (stammering something indistinct to herself).

T: "What did you say?"

P: "Why? Did I say something?" she sounds amazed.

T: "I saw you whispering."

P: "No ... I don't know ... I was thinking about my family."

T: "What do you mean?"

P: "I was thinking about my mother, in particular. They're losing faith in me and my abilities. They say that to me."

T: Not being clear at this point whether the patient is hearing voices or is reporting what her family usually says to her, I decided to opt for the second hypothesis and say to her, "Well, I think I've understood what you're telling me is that they are making financial sacrifices and expecting tangible results from you."

P: "What do you mean by tangible? They don't know anything about how I really am. They provide the money, but isn't that what parents should do for their daughter?"

T: "Really? Is this what 'parents' have to do?"

P: "Yes, but not just that ... [a pause]. But did she call you?"

T: "Who? Who do you think has called me?"

P: "My mum."

T: "Your mother? No, absolutely not."

P: "Ah, for a moment I thought she had sought you out. She does these things, she did it with my friends, she did it with my school teachers ..."

T: "I want to reassure you that I haven't received any calls from your family. I would be careful not to talk to them about what goes on in this room and particularly without involving you directly or having your consent."

P: "In any case, it is clear that they are interfering negatively in my life ... particularly now when I'm a long way from home."

T: "I don't understand. How are they interfering?"

P: "They are with me all the time ... this is the terrible thing about it ... she is always in my head! I can't stand it any more!" Silence. "She calls me every single day, she asks me what I'm doing, where I've been, what I'm studying, if I've eaten, etc., etc. The hell I'm studying. I'm studying all the time. Isn't that enough? I live in a big city and they have no idea what it's like to live alone in a big city."

T: "You're telling me that the fact that you are a loser has to do with geography? Do you want to go back to Italy?"

P: "So you really think I'm a loser?"

T: "Yes, of course. I can say it again if you want." Silence.

T: "So? You're not saying anything?"

P: "Well, I don't know what to say. You told me that I would feel understood here, safe." At this point, Alice appears to become mute, looking at me questioningly.

T: "When you say that perhaps there's something wrong inside you, I thought that was great. I think that today may be the first time that you've said something like that, that there's probably something 'off' in you. You always talk about what's wrong with your parents, your friends, your Alma Mater ... perhaps something is changing and I want to show that to you because psychotherapy is fundamentally about working on yourself."

This was certainly a difficult passage of our session, but I felt it was necessary to get her to admit she was a "loser" in order to help her acknowledge that something was "wrong" with her, that something psychotic was going on for her. In other words, that was how I managed to make her accept not only that she needed help, but also that she needed the permission to work more responsibly in therapy, and outside the therapy room, in order to improve her mental health.

As the clinical scenarios here show, work with subjects affected by paranoid psychosis can be particularly costly on a psychological level and sometimes risky on a physical one. On the other hand, there are patients, often in pre-psychotic circumstances, who respond favorably to empathic interventions aimed at encouraging greater self-esteem and counteracting experiences that are existentially precarious and do little for the integration of the ego.

These are patients who have found in paranoia both a rigid and fragile defense that provides them with some degree of psychic equilibrium. The internal fragility of the paranoid world is, in fact, sooner or later palpable to the therapist, as demonstrated by the quality of his or her anaclitic counter-transference in the therapeutic relationship with these patients.

Interbodily emotionality and corporealization

The problem that arises during work with more fragmented and barely differentiated cases of schizophrenia—that is, patients who mainly use schizoid-somatic transference within the analytic relationship—is basically one of method. And our method, as the poet Allen Ginsberg (1954) elegantly suggested, must be "purest meat"; it has to be living body, bargaining flesh in the relationship with the patient. The analyst's body is, therefore, irredeemably induced by the psychotic patient to bring itself onto the therapeutic scene and to communicate. Even the analyst's words undergo a transubstantiation and become flesh, little pieces and mouthfuls with which to nourish the primitive needs (which are not just oral) of the psychotic individual. At this primitive level of the relationship, the analyst is thus called on to take back ownership of his or her own protocol communication and to use his or her bodily countertransference as a "guiding tool" (Heimann, 1950) to understand the patient.

Bodily countertransference should be understood by therapists to mean using their own bodily self—in structural terms, their own Somatic Child (C_1)—in a conscious and systematic way, making available Adult parts of the personality (A_1, A_2) such as information about the affective-sensory experience that comes from their own body. This means that therapists have to recognize and experience, as part of their personal analysis and also through clinical supervision, their body as a sensitive extension of their psyche (complete with its history and traumas). This body is able to occupy a physical and therefore interbodily space, to perceive time thanks to time boundaries biologically inscribed in various forms of sensory experience, and to think by means of *e-motions* (namely, bodily actions charged with emotivity). From this perspective, experiences of psychotic fragmentation—even mutism and psychotic stupor, catatonia, stereotypical motor as well as verbal movements, and also other forms of bodily and emotional negativism in schizophrenia—are not proper "negative symptoms," as they are largely described in the official literature. "Negative symptoms" in psychotic processes *retain on the surface* the prolific marvels of the interior depths. They represent the indeterminate as well as real nudity of the unconscious and not-(yet)-conscious parts of the patient's psyche. As symptoms, they indicate something, and, more specifically, they signal the mystery, and even the dread, of the unknown, of the undifferentiated, of the Other—including the therapist—which is still a long way off being there and being formed in the patient's mind as other-than-self.

In work with patients affected by fragmentary psychosis, the analyst is quick—or at least so we hope—to notice the mismatch between his or her rational psychic activity and the materiality of his or her body, to the point where a contraction in the spoken register is often balanced against a radical expansion of powerful somatic-affective experiences and vice versa, as if one aspect cannot possibly coexist with the other. This echoes in the relational field the process of horizontal splitting within the patient. But it is precisely at this level of analysis of bodily-dissociative countertransference that the therapist actually experiences the schizophrenic individual's dissociative solutions. These are not conscious but charged with emotionality through displacement of the person's anguish of fragmentation into sensitive compartments of the analyst's own body or into specific organs. Lombardi (2016) referred to this peculiar aspect of countertransference in terms of transference *onto* the body: somatic countertransference corresponds to transference by the analyst onto their own body, which is a necessary condition for accompanying the analysands throughout the progressive approach to their own body (p. 35).

For example, during our sessions, Chris, the patient obsessed by the idea that his jaw had turned to stone (see section "Situating time in place or context" in Chapter 5), did not seem receptive to any of the more or less "intellectual" interpretations I offered him from time to time in an attempt to disentangle, and as a result try to explain, the reason for his unpleasant bodily sensations. Instead, in anticipation of our meetings, I became increasingly aware of a tension headache that could last for the whole day, only going away late in the evening. I began to feel more weary in general during the week, thinking between sessions about what was awaiting me and how I was physically only a few days away from seeing Chris again in my office. My verbal interjections during the sessions appeared to me to be increasingly repetitive and mechanical. It was as if my own speech had become more hesitant and slow and the content of what I was saying increasingly uncertain. Not only that, but my emotions seemed flatter, as if they had solidified, and I had the feeling that this analytic relationship would sooner or later become "petrified," just like an old cog, worn and slowly rusted inside with the passing of time.

But, in fact, it was the emergence of this distressing feeling of unbearable inertia that allowed me to make contact with Chris's similarly distressing anguish. And his anguish, although seemingly frozen in his jaw, was actually aimed right at me and our analytic relationship. It was an anguish that exposed the heaviness of my and his verbal transactions, their monotonous stereotypy, and it was probably anguish for an early end to the therapy and in a wider sense for an early psychological death. This type of emotional experience signaled a point of no return in Chris's analysis. Without the need to resort to new interpretations, within a few sessions we found an unexpected strength in the analytic relationship, as if we suddenly knew where we were going, where we would now guide our joint exploration.

With some surprise I was struck by Chris's provocations concerning the air that he breathed in my office, for example, when he said to me: "I feel like I'm in a birthing room here in your study, doctor." And, in fact, in the opposite corner of that large office, fortunately behind a closed curtain, there was actually a gynecological couch! At the time I could not afford the rent of another room that might have been more suitable for our psychotherapeutic work, perhaps in a more central area of London, and I was, therefore, in a shared office in which worked more doctors than psychotherapists. "You're right, Chris, psychotherapy is a bit like labor in a way, but sometimes one forgets how much one enjoys giving birth to children." We both guffawed. That was the start of a series of relational situations in which both Chris and

I gradually emerged from an almost fatal stasis, in which we both risked feeling "con-fused." Instead, we ended up making contact with specific and spontaneous aspects of our respective and different personalities.

Chris's case shows how the use of countertransference for therapeutic goals leads the therapist (although not immediately consciously) to make use of an *interbodily emotionality*, that is, feeling immersed in the experience of the body (one's own and other people's), to then be able to think—to follow Bion (1977 [1962])—with emotionalized bodies. This process is easier said than done. Nevertheless, what seems particularly useful from a methodological point of view is what the analyst does with his or her own body, or parts of it, to contain the unbearable emotions of the schizophrenic patient and therefore that person's unthought known, thereby accessing a protocol level of the therapeutic relationship.

Another excerpt from the clinical work with Abena, the young female patient I knew on the ward during her first psychotic episode, offers a paradigm example of this (see the section "Abena" in Chapter 4). As mentioned previously, during our first meetings on the ward, Abena spent the majority of her time in her room, remaining almost immobile in a curled-up position and stubbornly mute. This relational attitude of immobility and mutism only varied occasionally with sporadic verbalizations and motor stereotypies, to which it was almost impossible to give a clear connotation of thought or emotion. The patient's internal world was pervaded by an indecipherable undifferentiation that also contaminated my perception of my own identity. I felt myself to be increasingly flat and objectified, as if I too were just an ornament in the room, completely emptied of any social and even therapeutic role or function. At the time, my sessions with Abena formed disheartening and upsetting parentheses to my weekly clinical work. I felt like I was drowning in the chaotic and undifferentiated marasmus of pathological symbiosis where, nevertheless, something powerfully unconscious seemed to be going on *beyond* the symbiosis. This inexpressible certainly had something to do with my own and Abena's strenuous attempts to get out of that amorphous abyss as distinct personal entities (personalities), however little and multiple, like tiny bubbles in a vast ocean, infinitesimal voids closed in by a boundary, by a coherent limen, until they formed the beginnings of ego states that were more or less organized and distinct.

As our sessions went on, I found, with some surprise, a first point of novelty and differentiation within our relationship, specifically, in the way Abena interrupted her long silences by asking me in a stereotypical way, "So, shall we cut this quiff?" "Quiff?" I thought to myself, "what's all this about a quiff?" From time to time in this stereotypical transaction, which came up fairly regularly, I inferred something new: cut the quiff as an invitation to "climb down," that is, to be less arrogant; cut the quiff-penis as an attack by Abena on my virility; cut the quiff-tongue as a warning by her to say (or think?) less during the session; and so on. All were plausible interpretations, but thanks to regular supervision, I learned with effort to explain increasingly less to the patient. This was my way of *doing with her*: not making hasty interpretations, relinquishing any defensive maneuvers of rationalization, avoiding any verbalization of emotions or thoughts on behalf of Abena, and, instead, encouraging her own initiative and willingness to playfully explore new ways of being and interacting with me as the therapy progressed. I thus chose interventions, verbal and nonverbal, that were anaclitic. And to the umpteenth question of "so shall we cut this quiff?" one day I replied something like "would you like to touch it?" My invitation took the wind out of Abena's sails on a number of levels, as many as the number of plausible interpretations I had mentally worked over on the theme of "quiff." But after that something began to change in her attitude toward me. There appeared fleeting expressions of surprise, curiosity, smiling, and even wonder. These powerfully echoed the dimensions of play and exploration in which we are immersed when we relate to very small children but whom we treat as "adults in miniature" and thereby enable them to emerge as separate people from us. Resnik (2012 [1987]) appeared to reinforce this when he wrote, "The ludic sense of life, which is related to the idea of festival and of representation, and therefore to the theatre, is creative expression par excellence; the child that dwells inside each adult creates as he plays, by 're-creating' himself" (p. 195).

As the cases of Chris and Abena show, immersion in the experience of one's own body, often induced in more or less explicit ways by the patient, is translated into the analyst's hypersensitivity to certain internal perceptions (state of muscular tension, intestinal movements, heart rate, breathing rhythm, etc.) or even about how the therapist himself or herself looks and dresses. This can lead over time to functional neurovegetative symptoms (motor stereotypies, tachycardia, rapid breathing, etc.) and even culminate in actual physical disorders (muscular cramps, frequent urination, constipation, hypertension, etc.). On the one hand, therefore, the emergence (at times insidious) of bodily experiences risks getting in the way of the analyst's ability to mentalize; on the other, it allows the therapist to embody and share the polysensory and subsymbolic knowledge of his or her own ego-body and to communicate with the patient in a paraverbal and/or nonverbal register.

I call the latter process of embodiment of the ego *corporealization*. By this I basically mean grounding in the *reality of one's own living body*, that is, rebecoming "real" by means of a direct experience of one's own body. What makes this process problematic, however, is the ontological nature of our body. In fact, the body is par excellence the place of the Other. Like irreplicable otherness that is brought to life, we inhabit the body of the Other (from the intrauterine period of our development), and our body, from birth, is soon a place that is visited by the Other, a place of inexpressible passions and suffering, of boundless emotions, of primal images, of hallucinatory states and protomental actions whose course can bring us closer as well as distance us from the reality of successive preobject and object relationships. In other words, the nature of bodily-emotional states, established by patient and therapist through corporealization, is as transferential (relative to the very early relationships with the equivalent primary figures) as it is actual (relative to the here and now of the analytic relationship).

This is also why corporealization is almost never an easy process. In fact, it is a disturbing experience for the more mature and organized ego (particularly the therapist's) and consequently is accompanied by a plethora of defense mechanisms. Nevertheless, corporealization is necessary to bring us closer—or, rather, it brings us back to the transience of our being, to our insufficiency (and therefore irremediable dependency) as well as to the separateness of the Other (and therefore to our personal responsibility toward him or her or it). The body's grounding in reality is once again a process in service of the ego. It is probably one of the most arduous paths to follow for both the patient and the analyst; that is, to pass through the monodirectional mirror of primary exclusion (Berne, 1975 [1961], p. 61; see also Chapter 3 of this book). Corporealization, as a therapeutic process, is ultimately aimed at overcoming the experience of alienation left with the patient primarily by the traumatic void of the Parent-Other by inviting the therapeutic couple to a new relationality, to a mutual differentiation between self and other-than-self.

The body, in other words, is not only "living memory" (Resnik, 2005) but exists in the here and now and gives itself mutually in the relationship between therapist and patient. Contrary to Freud's assertions, rather than acquiring a primary pathological narcissism—which leads the patient to retreat into himself or herself, to autoeroticism, and consequently to a renunciation of the object world (including the therapist)—the psychotic individual reproposes through his or her body the current need for ontological recognition, which is required for the healthy narcissistic, and hence object, development of his or her personality. Formulated differently using Milner's (1987 [1977]) words, the presentation of the body on the therapeutic scene by the person in psychosis does not lead to "a narcissistic impoverishment of their relationship with the world, as you might expect, but, on the contrary, to an enrichment in this relationship" (p. 282). The specific existential condition of the psychotic individual—namely, fundamentally that of coming out as an individual "in pieces" in the relationship with the Other—is not enough to stop the tension of the ego in resolving this fragmentation by means of a somatic-affective relationship (C_1) with a new Other in the present (in particular, with the therapist).

In the same way, if viewed in terms of a recovery of the protocol register of experience, the therapist's corporealization is also not ascribed exclusively to countertransferential *enactment* of a narcissistic or even a fusional kind—and therefore erroneously ascribable to a certain type of pathological symbiosis—but becomes the therapeutic response to "yearning-for-the-Parent transactions" with which the patient unconsciously tries to actualize, beginning with his or her own Child ego state, the anaclitic needs that were historically unfulfilled.

Anaclitic transactions and bodily-emotional autoinduction

I previously described how anaclitic countertransference is the therapist's direct response to the "yearning" transactions for the primarily excluded Parent (P_1 or P_2) by the psychotic patient. However, because the primal exclusion occurs at a nonverbal protocol level of experience, anaclitic countertransference is the expression of nonconscious and unconscious activity of the therapist's Child ego state throughout development (C_2). Moreover, because of the traumatic (sometimes also objective) imprint of the relationship with the original Other, the anaclitic needs (which are irremediably infused with a bodily-emotional significance) that the patient induces via transference are paradoxically the same ones against which the patient herself not only strenuously defends but of which he or she (i.e., the patient) also has an acute nonconscious awareness. It follows that anaclitic countertransference too brings with it defensive distortions, which the therapist must know how to decode in order to guide the analytic process in a curative and progressive way for the patient.

The clinical experience I have gained through my work with psychotic patients and their families shows how the laws of intimacy—and therefore of love and hate, of life and death—are often hard and even cruel. However, they are also necessary for the growth of each and every one of us. These laws require the therapist to assume a deliberate interest and unconditional and long-term focus (*care*) on the patient, just as a good-enough parent would do for an infant or newly adolescent child. This implies that the therapist, in his or her guise as a good-enough parent, recognizes that he or she cannot know intellectually what "good enough" means in reality, thereby embracing a vocation for the indeterminate, for the unknown, and for the mystery of which the patient is the messenger in the analytic encounter. Laing (1959) firmly stated that "the main agent in uniting the patient, in allowing the pieces to come together and cohere, is the physician's [also meaning the analyst's] love, a love that recognizes the patient's total being, and accepts it, with no strings attached" (p. 165).

However, the cardinal difference between a loving parent-child relationship and that of the analyst-patient lies in the curative orientation of the latter. It is, in fact, the therapist's responsibility to gather together and satisfy the unsatisfied anaclitic needs of the patient through his or her anaclitic countertransference while at the same time avoiding ties of dependency and pathological symbiosis. The curative aspect of anaclitic countertransference in work with psychotic patients is as it is because it occurs within a specific relationship, the analytic one, and often requires long-term engagement, sometimes over years, particularly if carried out with patients who have a clinical history checkered with psychotic breakdowns.

With this in mind, Berne (1977 [1966]) talked about the kinds of intervention he deemed adequate, particularly in treating schizophrenic psychoses in the active phase: "Here the therapist may have to function deliberately as a Parent rather than as an Adult for a shorter or longer period, sometimes extending into years" (p. 248).

Outlined in the following paragraphs are the definitions Berne gave for each of these interventions—namely, support, reassurance, exhortation, and persuasion—which can be (re)considered here as actual anaclitic transactions in therapeutic work with schizophrenic patients. Alongside the definitions, I will also provide brief clinical excerpts that confirm the reality of Berne's observations.

Support: "This may be simple stroking, whose content, providing it is tactful, is irrelevant. Its effect may be enhanced if the content is appropriately permissive or protective" (Berne, 1977 [1966], p. 248).

What disturbed Mr Blake above all else, particularly at the start of our therapy, was my readiness to listen to him at length and, if I could actually have done this, even for hours. I intuited, and then he himself told me explicitly on several occasions, that a part of his ego rebelled at the proof that someone was interested in him, listening, with unshakable patience and interest, to all the stories he told about the Big Bang, planets in the solar system, the gods of Mount Olympus, and so on. He was profoundly "disturbed" by the unusual experience of being given all that attention to the point where his paranoid attitude began to encompass me too.

(P = Patient, T = Therapist)

P: "Don't joke doctor, I don't like this game."

T: "No joke." I watched him slowly calm down, but he stayed silent without saying anything further.

T: "I want to learn to listen to you. But at the same time I realize that this upsets you. I don't think you have many other people who really tell you how they feel when they're with you."

P: "Yes, I have no one." At this point he got up. He resolutely went to the door and before leaving turned and said, "See you tomorrow?"

T: "Are you sure you want to leave? I've still got time."

P: "No, that's enough. Better tomorrow."

T: "As you wish then. I will expect you tomorrow."

This clinical excerpt indicates how the transaction of support is therapeutic when the countertransference itself is congruent in its content with the anaclitic needs of the psychotic patient. In such circumstances, through transactions of support, whether spoken or silent, the therapist is able to maintain an emotional atmosphere in tune with the bodily-emotional inductions given by the patient.

Reassurance: "The Parental tone of voice may be more important than the content" and "it is hard for reassurance to fail if the patient's Child feels exposed" (Berne, 1977 [1966], p. 248).

Returning to the case of Chris, his principal somatic preoccupation relating to the "petrification" of his jaw had given me access to experiencing the same anguish, which might soon have left both of us without words to say and therefore without a future as patient and analyst.

Right in the middle of a session, while Chris was intent on staring at the floor between our two armchairs, I said more or less these words: "I wonder how it feels to speak without moving your jaw." I said this through gritted teeth, although managing to move my lips quite easily. Chris timidly lifted his gaze, and I continued, "Listen Chris, let's screw the jaw and become ventriloquists." Once again, we laughed uproariously together, discovering the possibility of turning to creativity and healthy humor every time Chris's anguish manifested itself in his jaw and in my head. This slowly alleviated our discomfort and instead expanded the repertoire of feelings and later also thoughts in our respective personalities. Through the physical impediment in his jaw, Chris and I accessed the anguish within our relationship, and Chris was ultimately able to be reassured and acknowledged in his emotions and his fundamental need to simply be himself.

This clinical scenario exemplifies how reassurance is therapeutic in contexts in which the intensity of the somatic-affective states induced in the therapist by the patient is significantly raised. In these situations, the therapist, starting from the bodily-emotional content of his or her countertransference, reassures the patient of the anaclitic value of the induced somatic-affective states, thereby containing them and reducing their intensity.

Exhortation as an intervention is both complementary to and, in certain cases, the opposite of reassurance: "Exhortation may in some situations produce gratifying results through compliance of the patient's Child" (Berne, 1977 [1966], p. 249).

To Abena, who provocatively suggested that she wanted to "cut the quiff" with the upturned point of my hair, I turned one day, exhorting her in just this way to approach and finally touch my hair with her hands.

(P = Patient, T = Therapist)

T: "So? Up you get, come here, and touch the quiff!"
P: Showing no hesitation and looking amused, she came toward me and placed the palm of her right hand right on the point: "Wow, it's really hard!" she said grinning.
T: "Why are you laughing?"
P: "No reason, because it's strange!" (continuing to laugh to herself).
T: "What are you thinking about Abena?"
P: "I'm excited."

What she meant by this was that she was sexually attracted to me, and she expressed this by letting out a series of spasmodic grins and giggles like an orgasm. The result seemed almost like a dramatized caricature and, in part, an enacted devaluation of her sexual desires and her perception of herself as an eroticized body. In this case, the anaclitic interventions targeted at Abena aimed, along with others, to exhort her to become both bodily and emotionally aware of sexual experiences, which she had partly repressed and, to a larger extent, had never actually tried to satisfy in a real relationship with a man. The theme of sexuality was just that, as she herself told me later, "a theme" and not an actual life experience because of her incredible fear of merging and "dissolving" completely in the sexual union with a man.

When correctly used, exhortation confirms the patient's anaclitic needs with the therapist clearly encouraging the intensification of the somatic-affective states induced during anaclitic transference. More generally, the goal of exhortation is to satisfy one or more developmental needs, facilitating in these patients progressive egoic maturation and individuation as a person. Berne himself noted, however, that one of the major risks of exhortation is reinforcing a dependent connection with the therapist. Particularly in work with schizophrenic patients, this can contribute to the reification of the therapist, namely, to the intensification of his or her feelings of omnipotence toward patients.

Persuasion "nearly always contains a strong element of seduction. ... The therapist should be sure he knows what the patient expects in return for his compliance and be prepared to deal with the ultimate consequences" (Berne, 1977 [1966], p. 249).

Persuasion is an anaclitic process that is particularly useful when the therapist is induced weakly by the patient to assume the role of a historical parent. This often occurs with paranoid patients when emotional induction experienced by the analyst in countertransference, if accepted, risks reinforcing the patient's splitting defenses and even intensifying his or her projective identification toward the therapist. In such situations, the difficult task of the analyst is to coax the patient into the same (pre)object state defensively projected onto the analyst himself or herself. These processes require a certain degree of therapeutic alliance so that the patient's "acquiescence" will permit the therapist to work on the patient's egoic integration. This "implicitly promised recompense" (Berne, 1977 [1966], p. 249) by the therapist corresponds to a progressive reappropriation by the patient of splitting projections that are injurious to his or her ego and that divide his or her significant others into good and evil.

Alice's case provides a clinical example of persuasion. Her frustration at not having sat any university exams enlarged her internal experience of being swallowed up and made powerless by a maternal *alter* (super)ego represented by the "mummy university." During our sessions, she decided that I too might be somehow controlled at a distance through telephone calls from her parents (specifically her mother) and that our analytic space was therefore also contaminated by that influence. The intervention reported here represents an attempt to persuade Alice to move the axis of observation onto herself and our relationship so that she could recover the power and responsibility of her

169

own perceptions and ultimately her way of feeling and thinking about a period in her life of ontological uncertainty and growing paranoia.

For example, I said, "The moment has arrived when we need to seriously consider that you are at the center of what is happening in your life, and I am here to be not only your mirror but to enter into your own arena, to confront with you your supposed enemies in the hope of ending this fight so that you can say good-bye to a series of spectators whom you feel right there inside your head and perhaps also perceive outside around you and who are waiting only to see you collapse into pieces." After a moment of silence, Alice replied, "I had never thought of psychotherapy as being something like this before."

Another situation in which persuasion is useful is when a patient needs a bodily-emotional experience that is not experienced by the therapist in his or her countertransference. These clinical scenarios are particularly common in analytic work with dissociated patients. The therapist may initially be summoned to a kind of bodily-emotional autoinduction through which he or she assumes, alternately, the preobject position of the patient as well as that of an ideal new parent. Because autoinduction entails a definite intervention by the therapist's Adult (A_2), autoinduced anaclitic countertransference may appear, at first, to be inauthentic or disjointed from preverbal experiences of the therapist's Child. For these reasons, if not helped by the Little Professor's (A_1) intuition, bodily-emotional autoinduction may not occur immediately. Delayed persuasion with respect to anaclitic needs that are expecting to be satisfied forms one of the "ultimate consequences" (Berne, 1977 [1966], p. 249) to which the analyst is exposed in these cases, that is, "paying a high price for not having provided it" (p. 249) earlier. Depending on the analytic work carried out and the quality of the therapeutic alliance, the price to be paid can assume a number of different forms, from breakdown, to interruption of the therapy, to mutual acknowledgment of one's own limits, as well as, in more successful cases, mutual dedication to the therapeutic process.

References

Berne, E. (1975). *Transactional analysis in psychotherapy: A systematic individual and social psychiatry.* London: Souvenir Press. (Original work published 1961)

Berne, E. (1977). *Principles of group treatment.* New York, NY: Grove Press. (Original work published 1966)

Bion, W. R. (1977). *Learning from experience.* London: William Heinemar. (Original work published 1962)

Bollas, C. (1987). *The shadow of the object: Psychoanalysis of the unthought known.* New York, NY: Columbia University Press.

Garfield, D. A. S. (2009). *Unbearable affect: A guide to the psychotherapy of psychosis.* London: Karnac Books. (Original work published 2005)

Ginsberg, A. (1954). *Collected poems 1947–1997.* New York, NY: Harper Collins.

Hargaden, H., & Sills, C. (2002). *Transactional analysis: A relational perspective.* Hove: Brunner-Routledge.

Heimann, P. (1950). On countertransference. *International Journal of Psychoanalysis,* 31, 81–84.

Kohut, H. (1971). *The analysis of the self: A systematic approach to the psychoanalytic treatment of narcissistic personality disorder.* New York, NY: International Universities Press.

Laing, R. D. (1959). *The divided self: An existential study in sanity and madness.* London: Penguin Books.

Lombardi, R. (2016). *Metà prigioniero, metà alato: La dissociazione corpo-mente in psicoanalisi.* Turin: Bollati Boringheri. [Translated into English (trans. unknown): *Body-mind dissociation in psychoanalysis: Development after Bion.* London: Routledge]

Milner, M. (1987). Winnicott and overlapping circles. In M. Milner, D. Tuckett (Ed.), *The suppressed madness of sane men: Forty-four years of exploring psychoanalysis.* London: Tavistock Publications. (Original work published 1977)

Racker, H. (1982). *Transference and countertransference.* London: Maresfield Reprints. (Original work published 1968)

Resnik, S. (2005). *Glacial times: A journey through the world of madness.* New York: Routledge.

Resnik, S. (2007). *Il teatro del sogno* [The theater of the dream]. Turin: Bollati Boringheri. (Original work published 1982)

Resnik, S. (2012). *The theatre of the dream* (A. Sheridan, Trans.). London: Routledge. (Original work published 1987)

Semrad, E., & Van Buskirk, D. (1969). *Teaching psychotherapy of psychotic patients.* New York, NY: Grune & Stratton.

8

THERAPEUTIC TRANSACTIONS

The body is much more than a mere biological reality or a "concrete original object" (Ferrari, 2004, p.48). It is also the substance of which our most primitive transactions are made—interbodily transactions—in relation to reference figures from our past. The Child within the Child (C_1) that Berne referred to is the psychic internalization of primitive interbodily states with one's first caregivers. Such an infantile Child (C_1) corresponds to a more or less coherent organization of polysensory experiences, unthought thoughts, nonverbalized emotions, and multiform behaviors and gestures in relation to the big Other of our prenatal, perinatal, and infant history. It is also for these reasons that interbodily experiences that find a structural representation in transactional analysis terms in the primitive expressions of the Somatic Child (C_1) have their basis in very early infancy and continue to survive and transform throughout the entire life course.

Therapy with psychotic patients passes through these deep layers of being, encountering distortions at a nonconscious level of relationship. The Child within the Child is also the forge from which the script protocol and subsequent palimpsest are formed, starting from body-to-body transactions (Mellacqua, 2014) with significant others from our past. C_1 is also the location of the fundamental distortions of our own self, which each of us carries inscribed on our (not necessarily repressed) unconscious. As a result, this is also the site of an individual's creativity and intuition as well as the original base from which the most pervasive pathological distortions of subsequent psychophysical development may arise.

For this reason, I consider bodily transactions to be a direct expression of primal protocol, that is, of the tissue level of experience. This level can lie dormant within us, although it can be reawakened through sensate experiences of the body. The body is, in fact—particularly in relationships with psychotic patients—a real "elephant in the room" that we tend to ignore or from which we defensively dissociate ourselves (as our patients do) to the detriment of true intimacy in our work and more generally in our relational life.

In this book I refer, in particular, to a subgroup of bodily transactions that can be used therapeutically, a group I call *e-motional transactions*. By using the adjective "e-motional," my intention is to legitimize the therapeutic use of these types of bodily transactions in a specific way in clinical work with psychotic patients. In other words, bodily transactions can be used clinically as e-motional transactions that are spoken and/or silent. These therapeutic transactions are endowed with a particular "motional" quality with its double meaning, particularly in the Anglo-Saxon sense of "moving"—that is, simultaneously "inducing movement or action" and "producing strong emotions."

First of all, e-motional transactions are indistinguishable in substance from classical "therapeutic operations" (Berne, 1977 [1966], Chapter 11) and, in many aspects, from "empathic transactions" (Hargaden & Sills, 2002, Chapter 8)—except, that is, for their source, which is almost exclusively the analyst's Child ego state, and their target, almost invariably the fragmented Child together with the nonintegrated Adult of the psychotic patient. They also differ in their notably "e-motional" nature—which means they are not only empathic—at a duplex level of producing therapeutic and emotional inductions in the other (as explained in Chapter 7 of this book).

Second, the choice to specify these therapeutic transactions with the adjective "e-motional" reflects the wider function that they play in endowing the patient's self with a renewed psychic structure—a sort of restructured Child ego state (C_2)—and consequently in inducing the psychotic ego to progress and develop toward more articulate and coherent forms of egoic integration (integrating Adult) as well as intersubjective differentiation (between self and other-than-self). This work of egoic structuring and restructuring—which paves the way for a more coherent experience (i.e., less fragmentary) of the individual's self and, thus, his or her individuation as a person—is deemed to be more effective in forms of schizophrenic psychosis when the ego already seems to have a better internal organization (e.g., late onset paranoid schizophrenia).

In summary, e-motional transactions exist in the sense that the patient does something to me and I do something to the patient but I, as the therapist, am responsible for sooner or later finding out how to report back to at least one of us—and preferably both—about what, in reality, we are doing to each other as our meetings go on.

For this reason, it is good for the analyst's Adult to remain (pro)active during the therapeutic process (helped, normally, by regular supervision), guaranteeing that communication between his or her Child and the patient's Child (or more than one, as in group therapy) is actually occurring and continues to take place during the therapeutic encounter.

In the following section, I describe three main categories of therapeutic transactions that I consider to be particularly relevant for transactional analysis of schizophrenic experiences: illustration, interpretation, and crystallization.

Illustration

Berne (1977 [1966], pp. 238–239) described the different types of illustration according to the role of the context in which they originate ("internal" or "external" to the analytic relationship) and the times when it is used ("immediate" or "remote") with respect to other therapeutic operations. When using illustration in analytic work with schizophrenic patients, it is important for the therapist to know what effect such an intervention will have on the patient's Child. In this regard, Berne noted how through illustrations the patient's Child allows itself "the freedom to laugh," the "freedom from literalness," and "permission for creativity" (p. 239). For these reasons, illustrations "should be humorous, or at least lively, and they should be intelligible to the Child of the patient as well as to his Adult; hence they must be couched in a vocabulary that a wise five-year-old could understand" (p. 238).

The use of illustration may, however, have effects that are not altogether therapeutic for the Child of the psychotic patient, depending on the structural pathology from which the person suffers. For example, in work with paranoid patients, Berne's recommendations to acknowledge a still-active role of P_1 (and in some cases also P_2), partially excluded, on the C_1 of the patient in these conditions are still valid. As a result, illustrations meant for a patient who resorts to persecutory-idealizing transference "may arouse more or less resentment in the Parent because of their obvious seductiveness to the Child, and such resentment will have to be dealt with sooner or later" (Berne, 1977 [1966], p. 239).

On the other hand, one should not ignore—particularly when using illustrations with the patient whose psychosis is dissociative—"the resentment in the [patient's] Child because they hurt his feelings, particularly in people who are collecting hurts, injustices, or tokens of their own inferiority" (Berne, 1977 [1966], p. 239). In the fragmented psychotic patient, the Child's resentment may take the form of either depression or a resurfacing of the anguish of fragmentation, both deriving from the progressive collapse of delusional beliefs (delusions) and the normalization of hallucinatory perceptions (disillusions). In these situations, injudicious use of illustrations by the therapist risks threatening the protection given to the Child—through the construction of delusions and hallucinations—by the excluded Parent (P_1 and P_2).

What follows is the elucidation of two types of illustration that are regarded as particularly useful in clinical work with schizophrenic patients: metaphor and allegory. These would be added to the patient's spontaneous choice (or encouraged by the analyst) to draw or paint as well as to use any other form of creative and artistic expression, such as poetry, music, and/or activities that can become the object of exploration in the analytic setting. In this book, however, we will focus solely on metaphor and allegory as examples of therapeutic illustration, leaving for future in-depth study the therapeutic use of creative artifacts that schizophrenic patients are often accomplished at producing.

Metaphor

Among the forms of illustration, metaphor is probably the most effective in recruiting the patient's Child at an emotional level. Language itself, said Umberto Eco (Eco & Paci, 1983), "is by nature, and originally, metaphorical" (p. 218). In other words, metaphor is certainly the true language of the Child. In clinical work with schizophrenic patients, metaphor is a therapeutic operation that the analyst can use for restructuring the Child, that is, for resolving the disorganization into which it descends because of processes of nonintegration and dissociation (emotional/bodily, emotional/cognitive, bodily/cognitive) and therefore egoic fragmentation.

Specifically, metaphor as a semantic tool enables, using few words, two things that are not immediately reconcilable on an intellectual level—and therefore not instantly comprehensible on an abstract level of thought—to be analogically juxtaposed. Metaphor is used, not always with awareness, to illustrate the meaning of something—for example, an external event, an intrapsychic process, a behavior, a physical sensation, or the reasons for an emotion or thought deemed to be intrusive by the subject—by using something else that makes the first thing comprehensible through the emotional participation of whomever shares the same metaphor. It is this emotional sharing between analyst and patient that facilitates an initial anchoring to reality shared in the analytic encounter and in the multiple meanings that this engenders.

My clinical experience with psychotic patients has allowed me to observe how in schizophrenia these individuals resort to metaphors about the body and in the register of the senses—whether through a subsymbolic (bodily) and symbolic nonverbal (imaginative, but not only this) channel—to substitute for a deficit in the use of a symbolic order, such as of a spoken kind that is more formal and abstract. Because recourse to the subsymbolic level (notably bodily) can be massive enough to absorb within it the imaginary and the activity of thought, emotional experiences and thoughts become concrete objects to the point where they form (as in the extreme case of catatonia) a freezing of intrapsychic and relational experience. Through the same process and in less extreme conditions, the Child ego state of the schizophrenic patient in breakdown risks stiffening and solidifying but also fracturing and dispersing its boundaries: words become food but also poison, thoughts are things but also weapons, the senses are receivers but also defenses, emotions become living flesh but also open wounds.

Metaphor is, therefore, a refined therapeutic tool with which the analyst can operate on the delicate boundary between the real and the imaginary, between what can be narrated in words (symbolic) and what requires narration through images (symbolic nonverbal) or even bodily, and between the conscious and the nonconscious (including the repressed unconscious). This consequently allows the use of a minimal verbal register to guarantee *healing by second intention*—that is, from the depths to the surface—of the split in many places (fragmentation) typical of the suffering in schizophrenia. I define this curative process as healing by second intention because—and it is worth repeating—the primary target of metaphor is the emotional recruitment of the deepest layers of the Child (C_1 and C_0) to facilitate a new, intuitive, (pre) verbal, and intersubjective understanding (A_1) from which shared and cocreated verbal meanings of experience may arise.

For example, Nathan, the patient distressed by the perception that his thoughts might end up sometimes in my bottle of water, gradually managed to claim back his projections and introjections precisely because of an intervention involving illustration based on metaphor.

(P = Patient, T = Therapist)

T: ": Nathan, you think that this bottle is a part of me and that I can steal your thoughts and close them up in here (showing the bottle), or that, in fact, I can make them disappear by swallowing them like air and water. ..."

P: "But what are you saying?"

T: "Do you perhaps think that I've drunk my own brain? Or even yours?"

P: "That's good," with a slight, tight smile.

T: "Perhaps it's why I see you sucking air when you sigh? Are you trying to stop your thoughts for fear that I will take them away?"

This explanation of what was going on—which we had reached through the recovery of a thought via metaphors instead of a thought via concrete objects—did not completely stop his sighs. And, although I had avoided drinking in subsequent sessions, even leaving the bottle open on the table behind me, Nathan continued to be obsessed with the idea that his thoughts could end up in that bottle. Nevertheless, something in Nathan's attitude toward me was changing: He began to be less suspicious in his interactions with me and more talkative until, following the metaphor of the bottle, he was able to talk to me about many other situations in which he had experienced the anguish of having his thoughts stolen to the point of "feeling read" in his mind. An example of this was all the times that the bus taking him to his destination had stopped exactly where he was standing, opening its doors right in front of his nose. Or those times when the math tutor at university called out "Be brave! Whoever knows the proof come clean or be silent forever," exhorting the students to speak out about a theorem that he already knew. Or the time his girlfriend, Helen, had unexpectedly kissed him and said to him seductively, "You're an open book to me, Nathan."

The ultimate aim of metaphor is to bring the imaginary back to the real, delusion to deliroid experiences, hallucination to illusion, the external world to the internal world (and vice versa), dreams to signs (or signals), madness to creativity—continuing the work of analysis until the apparent "enigma of schizophrenia" (Bollas, 2015) can find comprehensibility in the here and now of the transformative experience of the therapeutic relationship.

Thinking about it, this book itself is full of metaphors that use the senses and the body to describe particularly complex intrapsychic and relational processes of the schizophrenic experience and express them in a way that is immediate, hopefully without the need for long and boring explanations. In particular, the metaphor used by Berne to illustrate exclusion as a "one-way glass" (Berne, 1975 [1961], p. 66) formed a starting point to explain the structural psychopathology of schizophrenic psychoses from a perspective that arose directly from clinical practice. In truth, many metaphors that are particularly powerful on an emotional level—used by Berne and many other authors—refer back to the body, the five senses or physiological activities of the human (or animal) organism, in order to describe analytic and therapeutic processes.

Allegory

Allegory, like metaphor, belongs to the category of illustration. However, unlike metaphor, it consists of the intentional juxtaposition by the therapist of a signifier (i.e., a nonverbal symbolic object such as an image) and a signified (i.e., an object usually belonging to the register of the verbal symbolic). Allegory also recruits the patient's Child by acting at a (pre)verbal level that is both imaginary and intuitive (typical of A_1), but it leads to broader interpretative work. Through allegory, the therapist can introduce into the analytic conversation a receptive element of higher-level elaboration, and therefore of interpretation, coconstructed with the patient. From this we could say that allegory operates at an intermental level, which tends to be more intellectual, thereby taking the therapist and patient toward an exploration of the specific context to which allegory itself tends to refer (e.g., a family context, a traumatic event from the past, a work situation, a romantic relationship, etc.).

This tool is particularly effective in work with psychotic patients with a "hyperreflexivity of the self" (Sass & Parnas, 2003, p. 428), who tend to use rationalizing defenses, because it allows the therapist to attune horizontally with the patient at a cognitive level (A_1 and partly A_2) while continuing to stimulate in the patient vertical communication (intramental) with the most intuitive and emotional parts of his or her Child (still A_1 but also C_1).

Thus, we could say that, through allegory, the therapist targets healing by *primary intention*—that is, from the surface to the depths—of the injuries to the psychotic patient's Child. I define this curative process as healing by primary intention because the main target in this case is the active recruitment of the A_1 and the A_2 so that the somatic-affective "unthought known" (Bollas, 1987) information coming from the C_1 (through symptoms, memories, dreams, transference and countertransference enactments) can be progressively re-elaborated and integrated into an egoic organization (C_2 as well as A_2). This is more coherent as well as connected to a specific and real sociorelational context, past as well as present, analytic as well as extra-analytic.

On that note, I want to return to an exchange of transactions with Anisha. (P = Patient, T = Therapist)

T: "What happened to that book by Tagore that was on the shelf last week?"

P: "I've put it away."

T: "You've thrown it away?"

P: "Of course not! I've put it somewhere else."

T: "Where?"

P: "Where do you think I've put it? It's in here (indicating the trolley with the fingers of one hand)."

T: "Don't tell me you put books in the trolley?"

P: "And if I don't?"

T: "Well, I thought you used it for shopping."

P: "Shopping?" sniggering.

T: "Yes, shopping. Lots of people take one because it's easier than carrying bags up and down on the bus or underground."

P: "Well, I eat books, let's put it like that," she said with a self-satisfied look. At this we both laughed genuinely.

T: "OK, but where do you go with all these books?"

P: "Where does one go with lots of books in tow, Doctor?"

T: "Um ..."

P: "Do you know the Carnegie Library?"

T: "It's a bus stop."

P: "It's also a library."

T: "Ah, I see, and you go there to study?"

P: "I told you that people find it hard to believe me. You're like the others."

T: "It's because ..."

P: "No, please ... please ... I'm worried we'll laugh."

T: "Ok. I'm sorry, all right? I'm sorry. I have to admit that I have trouble, it's true, imagining you outside these four walls, out there as you say with other people around you." Long silence.

P: "There's no problem. I'm not by myself."

T: "What do you mean by not being by yourself?"

P: "I have my books, everything that is most dear to me."

T: "And perhaps that's why the other evening when I got in from work I thought about that book by Tagore."

P: "*Hungry Stones,*" Anisha added quietly.

T: "Precisely ... I saw something special in that title ... something to do with you, I think."

P: "Really?" she said to me curiously. And then she added, "What do you mean?"

T: "I was thinking about your situation today … I mean about your existential condition as well as the situation you're living in these days."

P: "And what do you think?"

T: "Well, perhaps it's not a thought … it's more an image of you … yes, an image of you, but also of you and me here in this room like hungry stones, hungry stones, hungry for something."

P: "Well, you can't judge a book by its cover." Silence.

T: "Well said. But perhaps that's exactly what I'm trying to ask you: If you wish to open a page of your story, if you agree to brush the dust off the book of your life and share something personal with me."

This little intervention of illustration marked a point of no return in our analysis. What Anisha subsequently shared were entire chapters of her life: the innumerable trips that she had gone on when she was younger, the different schools she had been to abroad, but also the many friendships that were interrupted and then lost due to her family frequently moving because her father worked as an Indian diplomat in a number of different embassies around the world. Listening to her, I seemed to see her entire life through images, finally seeing the truth in the poet Keats's (1931 [1819]) words, "A man's life of any worth is a continual allegory" (p. 327).

Even though allegory introduces a symbolic element in an intentional way—as demonstrated here with the deliberate use of the title, which was particularly suggestive in this case, of a book belonging to the patient—this intervention must stick to the principle of "economy of thought" (Berne, 1977 [1966], p. 239) typical of illustration. The aim is not to hold a philosophical or metaphysical discussion about the level of disorganization of the patient's Child, but rather to restructure the Child through the interposition of Adult elements based on giving the patient conscious responsibility for his or her own subjective experiences in relation to a specific real context. In the case of Anisha, the therapeutic objective was partly to make her aware of her isolated condition, how she had reduced herself down to an apparently dead weight, to a stone that was actually hungry for the Other, a stone that dust (an expression of the immobility of time) covered and at the same time showed and indicated its wish to be revealed and brought into the light.

In this sense, allegory can become a tool with which the therapist can work not only to stimulate the intentional thought of patients with regard to their own life experiences—whether in the past, present, or about the future—but also to reinforce their sense of identity, to protect them from the anguish of fragmentation and from a pervasive ontological insecurity.

Sensate interpretations

Among the therapeutic tools available to the analyst, interpretation is by far the best for targeting the core of psychotic pathology. In fact, if illustration through metaphor and allegory enables healing by secondary and primary intention of the wounds of the Child ego state (i.e., from the depth to the surface and vice versa), one could say that interpretation enables *healing by third intention*, that is, directly in the depths or, rather, from one depth to the next depth. In this way, it is slower but also more incisive and, fortunately, definitive because it is aimed at the structural pathology of the Child: "The Child presents its past experiences in coded form to the therapist, and the therapist's task is to decode and detoxify them, rectify distortions, and help the patient regroup the experiences" (Berne, 1977 [1966], pp. 242–243).

In the psychoanalytic tradition, beginning with Freud, interpretation is a tool with which the analyst brings out material repressed by the patient or, rather, makes conscious the patient's unconscious. For this reason, interpretative techniques relating to the unconscious content of the clinical material have a considerable rationale in the treatment of neurotic pathologies in which repression is deemed to be a psychodynamic mechanism—apart from anything else, one that is more developmentally mature in comparison to splitting—responsible for adaptations as well as the structural pathology of the neurotic ego. In contrast, the psychotic ego is an earlier ego, largely bodily, polysensory, preverbal, intuitive, and protomental, which has found in primal exclusion the fundamental solution (either paranoid or dissociative) to the incessant anguish of fragmentation arising from repeated relational traumas with the original parent (i.e. encoded in P_0, P_1, and possibly also P_2 ego states).

It is precisely on the basis of these indications that the decisive role played by *sensate interpretations* in the treatment of schizophrenic psychoses becomes clear. By sensate interpretation, I mean (re)construction by the analyst and patient of the patient's subjective experience (also in relation to significant others in his or her history and extra-analytical present) based on the feeling of reality (Federn, 1953 [1952])—in the first instance, the reality of this bipersonal (or pluripersonal) analytic experience as well as how it develops during the therapy sessions starting from the intersensory and interbodily experiences between the two (or more) participants in the therapeutic relationship. According to this assertion, interpretation in the treatment of psychoses is primarily a coconstruction of living material still in formation, not (or at least not at first) a (re)discovery of repressed material.

It follows, moreover, that sensate interpretation is, in essence, an interpretation in transference (rather than an interpretation of transference), and it consequently uses all the cognitive, emotional, behavioral, and bodily information experienced and dramatized (or interpreted) by the analyst in his or her actual countertransference (i.e., as the latter happens in the here and now of the analytic encounter). One might say, in the words of Bollas (2013), that sensate interpretation is not a question of intellect but rather has to do with a genuine "immersion in the material, in order that the mind can elaborate the encoded condensations through further unconscious work, laced with emotional experience and insights" (p. 86).

With paranoid schizophrenics especially, the action of interpretation can be undertaken by the therapist as both spoken and silent transactions. In the first case, it offers paranoid patients new perceptual choices according to their persecutory or omnipotent experiences with or without hallucinatory phenomena. In the second case, the therapist tends to use unspoken interpretations (i.e., not communicated verbally to the patient) in situations in which it is necessary to maintain an internal distance due to the intensity of experiences that are split and massively projected onto the analyst. It also offers the patient a tacit relational containment for his or her experiences of anguish. Moreover, silence provides the therapist with the necessary reflective space in which to formulate such interpretations.

In the following clinical excerpt, unspoken interpretations—as distinct from spoken interventions in the exchange between patient and therapist—are reported in square brackets.

I am again with Mr Blake. In the middle of a session during which the principal subject of discussion is once again his more or less unconscious obstinacy over wearing sunglasses even in the therapy room, the patient goes off again on his favorite refrain.

(P = Patient, T = Therapist)

P: "Helios, Hermes, Aphrodite, Gaia, Ares, Zeus, Cronus, Uranus, Pluto ... we are surrounded ... 136472 Make Make ... Make Love Make Love ... 136472 Where is the love? Stop procreation ... 136472 ... Where is the love? Stop procreation."

T: Silence [At this moment he is coming out of his body and fragmenting, his self-body has reduced into many fragments, projecting itself into distant space light years from this relationship; it has become a multitude of heavenly bodies, of bodies invisible to the naked eye, like his eyes, invisible because they are obscured. The fragments of his self exist only in the darkness of "interstellar space," light-years from us.]

P: "We are surrounded. Pluto, Uranus, Cronus, Zeus, Ares, Gaia, Aphrodite, Hermes, Helios ... 136472 Make Make ... Make Love Make Love."

T: "Why do you say that we are surrounded?"

P: Mr Blake: "We are surrounded. Where is the love? Stop procreation."

Because I do not have access to his eyes, my attention tunes powerfully into the acoustic channel as well as to my own and the patient's bodily sensations: to posture, breathing, voice. Mr Blake's tone of voice is rather harsh; the rhythm is particularly insistent, often interrupted by something that seems like loss of breath. As the session proceeds, I feel a state of muscular tension growing within me. My breathing also feels shallow, as if I might be about to do a warm-up before a workout or a race. I begin to register fear internally, a definite fear that finds in the patient's words "we are surrounded" almost a kind of acoustic reinforcement as well as an explicit confirmation of something distressing that now seemed to concern me personally. I therefore turned to another internal interpretation (silent) to deflect what I deemed to be, in that moment, a kind of projective counteridentification with experiences of strong anguish coming from the patient.

(P = Patient, T = Therapist)

T: Silence [You feel fragmented; you are reliving an original fragmentation; you are wondering where the sense of living, of loving, is, that perhaps it is better not to have been born, declaiming "stop procreation" in order not to have this frightening state of shattering, annihilation; you have a fear that is greater than you and that you are passing to me, yes, I feel it coming onto me, into me, but it is yours, only you don't know how to recognize it, take it back, or possess it.] At the umpteenth frantic repetition of the list of planets, I managed to give the following spoken interpretation to Mr Blake: "You want to escape from our meeting space, you want to lose yourself in the infinite space of the universe, where no one can see you with the naked eye; the planets are fragments a very long way from you, like your hidden eyes behind those dark glasses. You have found a way of going light-years away from others."

P: "Life has been unjust, cruel to me."

T: "Yes, this is why you wonder where the sense in living is, if perhaps it would be better to 'block births' because this life is full of anguish. You wonder where the sense of love is, if one comes into the world with a lot of suffering. And in all of these, I feel that you have a lot of fear. You are afraid that these planets that are fragments of you throw everyone to the ground, that they turn back and fall back on you, on us, killing us. You are not just talking about the origin of the universe. You are talking about the end of the world; you are living out an Armageddon. This therapy seems to you like an Armageddon, but I am here to find a new way out, but in reality, here on earth, not in interstellar space—in the reality that lives within you, not outside and a very long way from you, and which is known as the interior space."

As the sessions progressed, I made him aware of how a space existed that was as big and infinite as the interstellar one and that this space was the analytic space between him and me. I also tried to explain to him how this space was frightening for him because he feared me. The proof of this was his violent attempts to counteract my reflexive activity during the sessions by vomiting the list of his planets all over me. I told him also how it was not by chance that he had connected these planets with Greek gods who were anthropomorphic and often in battle with each other. I interpreted on more than one occasion how he was frightened of these planets because fundamentally they were a bizarre part of himself and unknown and "crazy" parts of others more generally. I told him, too, that it was likely that this happened because he had been frightened of significant others in his past, particularly his mother, who had been violent toward him but who was also seriously ill. I told him that, for fear of living like this, he had preferred the darkness to the light and that his dark glasses indicated this too and that I was not surprised when he told me once that he preferred going out at night rather than during the day, that "Brixton is more lively and colorful in the dark."

In addition, because, from a structural point of view, paranoid schizophrenia is viewed as more organized and developed on an egoic level, the therapist can initially stabilize the patient's Adult (A_1 and often also A_2) by offering explanations, comparisons, and specifications (Berne, 1977 [1966], Chapter 11). This work of stabilization and decontamination of the patient's Adult can also pave the way for work on the deconfusion of the Child based on more classical interpretations, such as those about content relating to repressed material (and therefore belonging to psychodevelopmental stages that are comparatively more mature) or interpretations of transference (which use extra-analytical, as well as historical, material talked about by the patient during previous sessions). It often arises in clinical work with paranoid patients that, even in those instances when interpretation has been accurate and offered at the right moment, the result does not always generate insight in the patient that resolves or ends the processes of splitting and projective identification. However, the effect, which can be seen through the progression of the analysis and through interpretative interventions, is a greater emotional resonance between analyst and patient. This emotional resonance leads to experiences that patients themselves register as precious because such instances are often rare for them: reciprocal listening and therefore real understanding of their own existential distress. In this way, patients can then be guided in a process of greater awareness of themselves, one that is based on reappropriation and progressive integration of the various parts of their personality that had been split and originally projected.

On the other hand, when treating dissociative schizophrenias, and in cases of less organized paranoid psychoses, sensate interpretation has the function of putting into words (Cardinal, 1983) experiences that are not only unconscious (because of defensive processes of vertical and horizontal splitting) but also nonconscious, that is, known but not yet thought, inarticulate and not yet verbalized because they were formed in early psychodevelopmental periods in the sphere of preobject relationships and protomental activity of the ego. In such clinical scenarios, the therapist finds himself or herself following a flow of the patient's psychotic experiences along with them, whether they are bodily sensations, images, or sensory experiences shared verbally or in silence (such as hallucinatory experiences) or delusional ideas and relational experiences that can be directly induced in the therapist or in which the therapist participates because of the powerful transference and countertransference dynamics. For example:

(P = Patient, T = Therapist)

183

T: "What's up, Nathan?"

P: "Nothing."

T: "Nothing is something though." Silence. "You are still staring at the bottle, which is open, as you can see."

P: "Yes."

T: "You're still worried about your thoughts?"

P: "I don't know. I think so."

T: "And what if it is just thirst?"

P: "Sorry, what? If I'm thirsty?"

T: "Yes, you. I wonder if you're thirsty, Nathan."

P: "You're the one who drinks in here."

T: "But it doesn't mean that you're not thirsty. And that perhaps you're also annoyed by the fact that I'm drinking and you're sitting there watching."

P: "Maybe a bit, yes."

T: "Because if you're thirsty you feel it, and it doesn't do to think about it. It is the same for the 'thirst' of your own thoughts, which I steal every time by closing them into this bottle. I would be very angry if someone stole my thoughts all the time; I'd be furious, Nathan, as well as scared. It's also true for me that I experience sitting here stealing your thoughts every time we meet as something very tiring as well as very depressing. Sometimes I wonder if you are also thirsty for thoughts that aren't yours, if you're thirsty for what I think and feel when I'm with you, if you're thirsty for what we each end up thinking and feeling about each other." Silence.

P: Then he adds uneasily: "I don't know. I mean at times it seems all confused. I don't know how I seem to you at times. But if you tell me that I'm angry. That is, I think I am, but ..."

T: "But?"

P: "I don't know. ...What shall we do? I mean if I'm thirsty as you say I am, but, I mean, there are also your thoughts."

T: "There you go, if you agree then next time you could get yourself a bottle of water. What do you think? Half a liter would do for a session?"

P: He looks at me incredulously, then adds, "Yes, to start with, half a liter would do."

This is how Resnik (2001 [1972], pp. 221–222) described the use of interpretation in the treatment of psychosis: I believe in transferential interpretation because it is precisely in this type of rapport that we can be witnesses to events. But, from the patient's point of view, it can happen that "I am not present at the session." Their transferential rapport happens in another place where I am not a witness. To follow the spatial "adventures" of the session at the level of transference means to recover the space and bring it back to the confines of the analytical framework in which the roles of patient and analyst can be formally identified, in a way in which the smallest alteration is evident and visible. If a patient alludes to their past and mentions, for example, that they were hit when they were small, the patient is referring to an experience that I was not witness to. But if I feel that the patient is punishing me with their words, in their way of talking to me, I would interpret this to mean that the child from the past is present in me and is being punished by him (by his words).

In transactional analysis terms, sensate interpretation gives the analyst—through a handhold by his or her Adult on the level of reality (including the reality of his or her own body)—a "real" immersion in the often dark and solitary abysses of the patient's madness in an attempt to facilitate a subsequent climb back up together, a climb of the analyst and the patient together toward the surface of the real or more light-filled horizons. In such cases, sensate interpretation is therefore acted, lived, and dramatized by the therapist in full with regard to the role that this specific relational situation assigns him or her within the analytic session.

For example, Nathan did bring a bottle of water to subsequent sessions. This soon became a part of him, his half-closed container of thoughts, sensations, and emotional experiences, his as much as mine, which he began to carry away with him and in him. Handling the obsession about his bottle in this way transformed it—also because of the work of sensate interpretations—into a need to quench the thirst, a primal thirst that had not been satisfied in his infancy and adolescence in relationship with his parents (who had separated after a period of bitter conflict when Nathan was around five years old). Associated with this thirst were emotions of hatred and desperation that had never before emerged into his consciousness and against which Nathan still defended himself for fear of the anguish of being annihilated by them. In fact, a phase of his analysis seemed to be complicated by the appearance of powerful projective dynamics of a persecutory kind toward me. His was fundamentally a thirst to be acknowledged in the legitimacy of his thoughts (and therefore in his identity as a thinking being) as well as to appear more or less "open" to aspects of his own egoic apparatus, which was still in (trans)formation. He needed to allow himself to "drink sips" (i.e., receive and assimilate slowly) the thoughts and emotions of Others who were emotionally important to him—including his actual parents and me—without drowning (i.e., without entering into "con-fusion").

As we can see, in analytic work with schizophrenic patients, it is not about being external and passive observers of the person's apparently meaningless or delusional experience (in the literal sense of "misleading") but about being active and present witnesses, coparticipants (i.e., willing and able to coparticipate in this experience) in the search to (re)find a common sense, to create the flow and thread of this shared experience, which continues to evolve in the here and now of the therapeutic relationship.

Crystallization

In Berne's (1977 [1966]) conceptualization, crystallization "is a statement of the patient's position from the Adult of the therapist to the Adult of the patient" (p. 245). With the particular condition of the nonintegration of the Adult of the psychotic individual—coinciding structurally with a traumatized A_1 and an insufficiently organized A_2—crystallization aims to give (or repeat) information to the patient's Adult as well as to inform the Adult. This introduces a transformative principle that allows the Adult to implement a progressive (re)organization, and, as a result, integration and differentiation of the ego. In this way, in work with patients in psychotic breakdown, crystallization may be used in initial phases of the therapeutic process as well as subsequently alongside the interventions of illustration and interpretation.

When used in the middle of a psychotic breakdown, crystallization feeds the patient's Adult need to know what is happening to him or her, why whatever is happening concerns him or her directly, and what can be done to change the situation. For patients in crisis who are struggling with bodily-emotional experiences that are so intense that they are beyond the rational control of the Adult (A_2), crystallization acts as a dam to the imminent anguish of fragmentation and provides reassurance by offering an intellectual overview with which the person can see the experience of his or her own self from a less disturbing perspective. In such cases, crystallization assumes the form of an explanation and enables the therapy contract to be better formulated on the basis of the information gathered to that point about the patient's history, the type of structural pathology from which his or her Child is suffering, the analysis of the first transference and countertransference enactments, and the nature of the interbodily experiences that are protocol-based in their essence.

I return here to my clinical work with Alice, the young Italian university student enrolled in a degree course in history at King's College in London after a failed year at Bologna in the faculty of law pursuing her initial idea to become a criminal lawyer as her maternal grandfather and mother had been. At a certain point in the analytic work, Alice insisted again on tracing back the difficulties with her studies—and, to an extent, with the therapy—to the negative influence of her mother.

The session described here follows a brief interruption because of the Christmas holidays. Alice went back to Bologna, mainly to, in her words, see her school friends. Her parents were divorced and her father had lived in France with a new partner for about two years. Alice said she spent barely a day in the company of her mother despite being at home with her. She confided to me how during a dinner at home with her mother, Alice was struck with the alarming thought that her mother had somehow tried to "poison her" by spiking her wine with drops of a sedative. Although Alice believed this thought to be mostly "bizarre," she admitted to having deliberately turned down all subsequent invitations from her mother to meet even after Christmas, ultimately describing the days spent in Italy as filled with deep discontent and inability to concentrate on her studies.

At the time of the session described here, Alice felt confused but not tired and said she was incredibly behind with essays due for her course in medieval history.

(P = Patient, T = Therapist)

P: "I've had enough of telling you what I'm thinking. I think I'm wasting precious time coming here. I just need to study. Here I'm just wasting time, time."

T: "Study doesn't preclude the analysis, Alice."

P: "Here I feel confused … too many events from my past are coming out here; I have already wasted time, going on like this I become the loser in everyone's eyes, not just my mother's or yours."

T: "Alice, what do you intend to do then?"

P: "Study nonstop. I must succeed this time, whatever the cost."

T: "Don't you think you're already paying a high price by how you're living out your days?"

P: "Perhaps, but that's your opinion and you could be wrong."

T: "Of course. I can't read the future, Alice. But yours seems to be going stubbornly in one direction."

P: "I just have to shake off this negativity crap that is dogging me." A long silence follows. Then Alice resumes the conversation and, with eyes full of tears, adds in a low voice, "I don't understand anything any more, doc, I'm going mad."

T: "The difficulty, Alice, is not in understanding. You can't understand everything straightaway. Your real difficulty, or even your tragedy, lies in you not wanting to feel what your emotions are expressing, in you not wanting to see what your body is showing you. You continue to maintain that you don't have time, and your way of throwing yourself into your studies enables you not to get in touch with all the frustration and all the hatred that you feel for your family, particularly your mother, hatred that you instead attribute to your mother rather than to you. This increasingly threatening role, which you give to your mother, you are now also giving to me and this therapy. This is creating flaws in your way of thinking, and there are signs that your thoughts are taking specific paths that are difficult to follow on the level of reality. And then, look at yourself, see your body becoming thinner and your face paler. All this is happening to the detriment of your needs: like that of being accepted for who you are and being loved despite your more genuine ambitions and despite the limitations and frustrations that you are encountering in your life."

From this crystallization, a more contractual phase of therapy with Alice began. Our sessions proceeded with a regular flow of once or sometimes twice a week for three years or so. Alice got her degree in history and decided to pursue academic studies with the aim of undertaking a research doctorate in medieval history. In one of our final sessions, Alice looked back over her therapy and saw a progressive emancipation from persecutory experiences that revolved mainly around her relationship with her mother. She had been learning to negotiate with these aspects of her internal and relational world and to integrate them, rather than believe them to be completely alien to her: "Just like in medieval times," she said to me, "when the barbarian invasions gradually gave way to the constitution of feudal lordships and the first communities."

In work with schizophrenics with a more disorganized ego, crystallization acts, in addition, as an "alpha function" (Bion, 1977 [1962]), and better still, as a "transitional mental object [through which] the self is now being instructed from within" (Bollas, 2013, p. 88). It helps the patient's Little Professor (A_1) learn, over time, about the workings and sensate experiences of his or her bodily ego (C_1)—emotions, anaclitic needs, fantasies, dreams—as well as about the toxicity and interference of his or her traumatic original Parent (P_1). In this way, wrote Berne (1975 [1961]),

> When a[n] ... archaic ego state is revived in its full vividness in the waking state, it is then permanently at the disposal of the patient and the therapist for detailed examination. ... [Then] the [patient's] ego state can be treated like an actual child. It can be nurtured carefully, even tenderly, until it unfolds like a flower, revealing all the complexities of its internal structure. It can be turned over and over in the hand, so to speak, until previously unobserved features come into full perception
>
> (p. 226)

The following is an example of that process with a patient named Sally.
(P = Patient, T = Therapist)

P: "I'm better."

T: "I can see that, Sally."

P: "But they have taken away our son."

T: "Our son is still alive."

P: "You allowed him to be taken away."

T: "What you call 'our son' is a fantasy, Sally. It is a fantasy that is still so vivid as to seem real, precious, and fragile, like a newborn. 'Our son' is us, 'our son,' as you call him, is the conception of these encounters, it is this relationship, it's what we are taking care of together. You have spent days walking in bare feet around this room in silence, wanting to control but at the same time indicating that there is a void that you have carried inside for who knows how long. I have penetrated this void with my steps, over and over again, our faces have met and then came the words. You have hated me and part of you still hates me for this unexpected intimacy. You have felt violated inside. You are scared of your void and try to limit it because ultimately you know that fertile voids do exist and that the void can suck in others, and now you know too that from the void can also come fantasy, emotions that possess us from the inside and in our bodies. From the void are also born images of dreams and even obscene words that another part of you does not want to hear or say. As long as you take a hand in controlling or even suppressing this void, maybe you won't write your poems and your stories again as you did when you were younger. You will go around barefoot in isolated places, like this hospital room, as if you were a nun in a convent, physically and mentally distant from other people, from the world."

Sally registered every single sentence of my spoken intervention, but she took weeks to digest it. She accused me openly of having raped her, of having abused her emotionally, of having flushed out her brain, before admitting to herself and then also to me that I was right about one thing: that she hated me deeply. Only a long time after, as our sessions progressed, "it came to light" how this hatred originated, among other things, from elements of her unconscious that were still not clear to her and that related to traumatic relational experiences from her past. These included, for example, the prudish and hypermoralizing Catholic teaching that she had received from her Irish mother and grandmother, the terror of losing her virginity because of constant fear of permanently losing the emotional ties with the only female figures in her past, her first homosexual experiences with a university colleague to avoid even friendly relationships with men, and so on.

When crystallization is used over the entire course of therapy, its clinical aim is to keep open a gap of awareness (breakthrough) in the developing Adult (A_1 and A_2) of the schizophrenic patient until it creates a true opening toward his or her Child self, transforming its fractures or wounds into "fissures" through which to look after traumatic, and still vivid, experiences from the past.

In conclusion, to use a surgical metaphor once again, consistent with Berne's style of writing, we could say that crystallization is like a therapeutic operation of "packing" and, at the same time, "draining" the deep wounds of the Child ego state, thereby enabling it, as happens with interpretation, to heal by third intention.

References

Berne, E. (1975). *Transactional analysis in psychotherapy: A systematic individual and social psychiatry*. London: Souvenir Press. (Original work published 1961).

Berne, E. (1977). *Principles of group treatment*. New York, NY: Grove Press. (Original work published 1966)

Bion, W. R. (1977). *Learning from experience*. London: William Heinemar. (Original work published 1962)

Bollas, C. (1987). *The shadow of the object: Psychoanalysis of the unthought known*. New York, NY: Columbia University Press.

Bollas, C. (2013). *Catch them before they fall: The psychoanalysis of breakdown*. London: Routledge.

Bollas, C. (2015). *When the sun bursts: The enigma of schizophrenia*. New Haven, CT: Yale University Press.

Cardinal, M. (1983). *The words to say it*. Cambridge, MA: Vanvactor & Goodheart.

Eco, U., & Paci, C. (1983). The scandal of metaphor: Metaphorology and semiotics. *Poetics Today*, 4, 217–257.

Federn, P. (1953). *Ego psychology and the psychoses*. London: Imago Publishing. (Original work published 1952)

Ferrari, B. (2004). *From the eclipse of the body to the dawn of the thought*. London: Free Association Books.

Hargaden, H., & Sills, C. (2002). *Transactional analysis: A relational perspective*. Hove: Brunner-Routledge.

Keats, J. (1931). Letter to George and Georgiana Keats, 14 February–3 May 1819. In M. B. Forman (Ed.), *The Letters of John Keats* (Vol. 2, p. 327). London: Oxford University Press. (Original work published 1819)

Mellacqua, Z. (2014). Beyond symbiosis: The role of primal exclusion in schizophrenic psychosis. *Transactional Analysis Journal*, 44, 8–30.

Resnik, S. (2001). *Persona e psicosi* [Person and psychosis]. Turin: Einaudi. (Original work published 1972)

Sass, L. A., & Parnas, J. (2003). Schizophrenia, consciousness, and the self. *Schizophrenia Bulletin*, 29, 427–444.

9

DREAMING REALITY

The transactional analysis interpretation of dreams

Berne's (1969 [1957]) seminal considerations regarding dream phenomena and their interpretation clearly originated in the psychoanalytic model of dream analysis presented in Freud's (1953 [1900]) groundbreaking *The interpretation of dreams*. Indeed, in Chapter 4 of *A layman's guide to psychiatry and psychoanalysis*, Berne (1969 [1957], pp. 129–136) confirmed Freud's view that people's dreams are open doors to their unconscious life and that we need the dreamer's free associations in order to interpret the dreams meaningfully. Formulated in Berne's terms,

> dreams are wish fulfillments in disguise. We have seen that it is necessary to obtain the dreamer's associations in order to interpret a dream properly, and that such interpretations reveal the dreamer's unconscious wishes to such an extent that dreams have been called "the highroad to the unconscious."
>
> (p. 135)

Earlier in the same chapter, in an effort to present the contents of the unconscious to the reader, Berne (1969 [1957]) offered a powerfully succinct yet systematic theory of the unconscious and its close relationship with the non(yet)conscious and external reality:

> The contents of the unconscious consist mainly of the "unfinished business of childhood" and matters related thereto. This includes tensions which have never become conscious, but are still capable of influencing behavior indirectly, and tensions which were once conscious and have been repressed. Together with these tensions are found the corresponding images: some which have never become conscious, and others which have been pushed out of consciousness.

Since imaginings, or fantasies, are just as real to the unconscious as actual experiences, many of the representations in the unconscious have little connection with reality, and yet are just as influential as realities.

(pp. 127–128)

To summarize, in Berne's initial formulation, dreams maintain a link with experiences of the individual's mental life and life experiences that are largely non(yet)conscious and/or unconscious (as a result of defensive mechanisms and survival decisions).

In addition, the concept of tension (or wish) in *A layman's guide to psychiatry and psychoanalysis* (Berne, 1969 [1957]) never appears to be an exclusively intrapsychic and solipsistic event freed from the object relation matrix of its genesis. This is clearly illustrated in Berne's description of Mr Meleager's dream (pp. 129–136) and introduces us to Berne's subsequent, more object-related view of dreams.

A second theory of dreams from Berne, closely related to the one just described, can be found in *What do you say after you say hello?* There Berne (1975 [1972], pp. 202–205) introduced the idea of the *script-set dream* and presented dreams in terms of images of a fairy-tale world that are also rooted in early childhood. What is particularly significant in this later view is the pictorial nature of dreams, which allows for a powerful reorganization of one's experience in relation to self, other (therapist included), and the world in general: "The 'script-set dream' is recognizable because as soon as the patient tells it, many things fall into place. Pictorially, it has no resemblance to the patient's actual way of life, but transactionally, it is an exact replica" (p. 204).

According to this view, a patient's dream can be seen as a reenacted drama—through transference-countertransference (i.e., through the analysis of basic positions, ulterior transactions, racket feelings, and games)—of his or her script protocol and script scenes in the here and now of the analytic session.

The epistemological foundations of this approach stem from Karl Abraham's (1955 [1909]) work on dreams, myths, and character formation as well as from Melanie Klein's (1975 [1961], 1997 [1932]) approach to dreams and play in child analysis. In Klein's perspective, in particular, the patient's dream is reminiscent of early phantasmatic life and is based on unconscious fantasies originating in early relations with primary objects. Fairbairn (1952) also followed along similar lines with his theory about how the mind works when producing dreams. He considered dreams to be dramatizations of various parts of the dreamer's internalized objects, which take the form of characters, scenes, and actual object relations (including the analytic relationship) that together reflect the actual state of the patient's inner as well as relational world.

In truth, Berne's (1969 [1957], pp. 129–136) section in *A layman's guide* on "Why do people dream?" contains a much less developed third theory about dream formation and the functions of dreaming. It purports that dreams "have another function, and that is to assist in healing the mind after emotional wounds and distressing emotional experiences" (p. 135). This is clearly illustrated in Berne's description of the case of Mr Simon Siefuss (pp. 169–172), in which a recurring posttrauma dream of a war veteran is worked out by means of a rather peculiar methodology. Indeed, this approach seems to involve far more active participation by the analyst in "living out," rather than interpreting, the pent-up tensions embedded in the patient's nightmare so that they can first be enacted in the presence of a new significant other, then released, and finally relieved.

More importantly, in the same section on "Why do people dream?", Berne (1969 [1957]) added, "Even ordinary emotional experiences have to be 'digested' in some way through dreaming in order for the individual to feel well" (p.136). This view on dream functioning suggests that the dream is not only the protector of sleep (Freud), but it also has a "digestive" function that is necessary and healing. Here, interestingly, Berne seemed to anticipate Bion's (1977 [1962]) much more influential distinction between what he called the *beta-* and the *alpha-elements* of mental life: the beta-elements—that is, raw "sense-impressions related to an emotional experience" (p. 17)—that reach symbolic representation in a dream become thereby thinkable experiences and reflective thinking, which are alpha-elements.

All things considered, the technique of dream interpretation, specifically in clinical work with schizophrenic patients, requires further epistemological and methodological consideration.

Dream analysis in schizophrenia

To approach the topic of dream analysis in schizophrenia, I will necessarily refer to my clinical work on dreams with psychotic patients. However, before looking in more detail at the clinical material, I will first return to Berne's more methodological considerations in relation to dream interpretation and from there explore how direct clinical practice can further inform transactional analysis theory as well as enrich its methodological approaches to dreamwork with schizophrenic patients.

First, in line with a "classical" (i.e., Freudian) technique, Berne (1969 [1957]) believed that the purpose of dream interpretation is

> to find out which Id tensions are trying to find expression in the dream, their true aims and objects, and their meaning for the individual. These factors are called the "latent content" of the dream. The dream itself, as the dreamer experiences it and tells it, is called the

"manifest content." The interpretation is an attempt to trace back from the manifest content to the latent content.

(p. 136)

Despite Berne's explicit suggestion to disentangle the manifest content (i.e., the account given by the patient of his or her dream) from the latent content (i.e., to some extent considered a more genuine expression of the patient's unconscious mental life), my practice of dream analysis with psychotic patients seems to have followed a different path. For example, consider the following dream from Chris, the patient described earlier (see Chapter 5) who was distressed by his "jaw of stone." Although Chris had not been able to recall his dreams for several years, as the analysis progressed he began to dream again. In particular, the dream described here shows, both iconically and laconically, his ambivalence toward the change that was happening to him during the analysis.

> I'm lying on a rigid dental chair. The air I'm breathing is very humid, and I can see steam in the corners of the room. A very young man with a pale face and dressed all in white, who reminds me of my childhood dentist, approaches to give my mouth a thorough inspection. He tells me to close my eyes under the blinding light. On his command, I open my mouth with difficulty. I do not hear the usual sound of the drill, which makes me tense up every time, but instead an unnatural silence that makes me open my eyes. Just above my nose I see an enormous white fork piercing a steaming yellow dumpling. I am literally stunned by the sight. In a trembling voice, I say to him, "Hey wait, what's this about?" The dentist states that my disease has nothing to do with my jaw. "What's with the dumplings then?" I ask in anguish. But his answer is, "Eat, these are made of fresh pasta and meat."

The substance of Chris's dream was structured as dreamlike language that primarily revealed a kind of hypersensitivity of the dreamer to sensory experiences: the blinding light in the room, the white color that dominates everything from the dentist's clothing to the pallor of his face to the color of the fork that he is holding and the clear contrast with the yellow of the dumpling, then the humidity and steam in his surroundings, the unexpected silence, and so on. This image of Chris—as someone with particularly heightened senses—contrasted with the hyperrationality and dulled emotional response he showed during his analytic sessions.

In addition, and even more interestingly, Chris maintained at the start of his analysis that he had been developing a genuine obsession with his jaw for about a year. But it was this dream that enabled him to recognize, among other things, how even as a child he had been troubled. The man dressed in

194

white in the dream actually reminded him of his childhood dentist. At around age five, Chris developed a stutter for which his parents had to enlist the help of a speech therapist. The stutter was resolved but then reappeared in a less striking form during adolescence.

Ultimately, taken as a whole, the dream illustrated a demolition of Chris's hypochondriacal fantasy relating to his jaw. In fact, his mouth even trembled at the idea that the problem of his psychic malaise was not his jaw, in the same way that it was not in his head (i.e., the location of intelligence). Rather, it was in something that lay somewhere in between, suspended in the air like the dumpling in the dream. The somatic delusion—to some extent unconsciously defended by Chris as a pseudoscientific hypothesis to explain his own schizophrenic condition—offered him only the appearance of a unified ego. It was that broken-down jaw that moved in jerks that always interrupted the harmony of his sense of being unified. Within the laboratory of the analysis (i. e., the dental studio of his dream), the ego discovered a false problem (the jaw) and then rediscovered, through the massive recovery of the senses, his own "meat," his own affectivity, "filled," just like a dumpling, with anguish for his relationship with the Other.

This clinical excerpt indicates, on a theoretical level, how Chris's manifest dream overlapped, de facto, with the dream's latent content, partly by corroborating a more general view within transactional analysis that dreams are expressed, in large part, through the language of the Child ego state (Tangolo, 2015). In other words, the dream as Chris told it appeared to be a direct expression of his Child self and, as such, was articulated using a different language, one that required translation rather than interpretation. This language was, in fact, internally structured as a narrative dominated by the senses and primarily experienced at a bodily-emotional level. It is also possible to develop (or not) the narrative into a visual scene populated by characters (i.e., internalized objects/Others and part-objects/part-Others). This language could also be represented as an anonymous scene with physical and only apparently inanimate objects, places, elements of nature, animals, and so on, but each in search of a single author (i.e., a more coherent sense of the self).

Thus, this first methodological approach to dream analysis with psychotic patients appears far more congruent with Berne's (1969 [1957]) clearer explanation of what it truly means to "interpret" a person's dream:

> It is a common error to suppose that *finding out* the meaning of the dream is the important thing. This is not so. The meanings must be felt, and these feelings must be put into proper perspective with other past and present feelings of that particular person, for the interpretation to have any effect in changing the underlying Id tensions, which is the purpose of the procedure.
>
> (pp. 136–137)

In other words, I suggest that what Berne defined as latent content stems from the emotional experience that a particular dream by a psychotic patient is trying to convey in the here and now of the analytic relationship. This emotional experience, embodied in the narrative and prosody of the patient's dream, might have a strong resonance with the past of the patient and, at times, with that of the therapist, although it is not necessarily or exclusively linked to traumatic memories. More importantly, in line with these considerations, the patient's dream takes the form of a new bodily-emotional experience that both patient and therapist can take part in, thereby actively contributing to a coconstruction of new meanings.

Berne (1969 [1957]) suggested a second methodological step to the analysis of dreams when he wrote:

> The interpreter bears in mind that the dreamer writes his own scenario. The dream is the sole product of his individual mind. Like the author of any scenario, he can put in any characters he pleases and do with them as he will.
>
> (p. 138)

This means, however, that the analyst can be actively recruited (as well as "disguised") as a character in his or her patient's dreams. That is to say, the patient's scenario tells as much about the patient as it does about his or her relationship with actual significant others, including the analyst. Less obvious than it may appear, this is very much the case in dream analysis with psychotic patients.

Following on from this, I will now describe a dream had by Alice, the young patient who had left Bologna and moved to London to take a new degree course in history (see also section on "Situating time in place or context" in Chapter 5).

> Last night I had a strange dream. I'm at my parents' house, and I'm in the kitchen. I sit helplessly at a corner of the table with my head in my hands while my mum and dad are in the midst of yet another violent quarrel. Around me is just noise: screaming, crying, slapping, spitting. The telephone rings. I go into the living room and pick up the phone. I hear the voice of a man who speaks to me, but I can't work out what he's saying. I can only make out that it's about my older brother. But I don't have any brothers. His voice is reassuring even though I cannot hear what he is saying to me. There is too much noise in the house. I quickly write down on a piece of paper "Tuesday at 7:30 p.m." I leave the house and mentally repeat "casa" (house), "caso" (circumstance), "oc-casi-oni" (occasions). I wake up with these words going round in my head.

While Alice was recounting this dream to me, I was immediately struck by the general acoustic sensory quality with which she was (re)living the dream scene. I also realized how the dream paralleled us and the noises in our therapy room. Alice was, in fact, mute in her dream, unlike how she was in our sessions where she was actually remarkably talkative. Furthermore, in the dream she appeared to be enveloped in sounds such as shouts, violent blows, and crying. Similarly, auditory hallucinations in the form of indistinct sounds and "voices in her head" intruded from time to time in her internal world, distracting her from the surrounding environment and her relationship with me. Once again, the sounds risked becoming a substitute for dialogue. Her head was bowed over the table, and it was often also that way during sessions. But Alice was listening more attentively than she seemed to when she was awake. She was telling me, with her dream, that she was listening. Nevertheless, we still did not know anything of her emotions, about how she was feeling in her heart, her stomach. But my voice was unexpected and reassuring, like that of an "older brother" that she never had. This voice reached inside her, it penetrated the family's chaos and took her away from the home, transforming the unforeseen "caso" (circumstance) of actually being at home at that moment—as well as, more generally, being born into that family—into an "occasione" (occasion) to leave and meet someone else away from the house, away from the chaos toward a new intimacy. "7:30," as Alice herself acknowledged immediately after recounting her dream, was the usual time for our sessions, although we met on Thursdays, not Tuesdays.

Here we find, in essence, a second perspective on the methodology of dream analysis in schizophrenia (not only in schizophrenic disorders). This method understands dreams as the representation of the here-and-now transference and countertransference in the analysis. We are, therefore, operating once again in the terrain of the unconscious, with its tensions being represented in dreams as "unfinished business because they have not yet been relieved, do not disappear until they are relieved, and are continually seeking complete or partial relief through their true aims and objects or through substitutes" (Berne, 1969 [1957], p. 128).

By analyzing the dream together, Alice and I acknowledged how the quality of our relationship in the analytic setting had reached a turning point. I had been actively recruited by the patient's unconscious and allowed to act as an unexpected "older brother" (even though the patient was an only child). From then on, and for most of our therapy, I became a newly needed Other, able to "meet" Alice and share and finally overcome together her terrible emotions in the midst of her recurring crises. We may say that dream analysis, from a more object-related perspective, serves a much larger purpose, namely "creating a containing human context in which the patient may be able to live with his past and present emotional experience (as opposed to evacuating it or deadening himself to it)" (Ogden, 2005, p. 21).

Once established, psychosis tends, among other things, to dehumanize life. It does so by displacing physical sensations, emotions, images, and thoughts from the person's inner world and moving them elsewhere and by impoverishing relationships with others, weakening intentions and social behaviors. In the most tragic circumstances, psychosis reduces the individual's existence to nothingness. It leaves him or her with no apparent history of intimate relationships and therefore with no intimate story to tell. But, as with Alice, psychotic patients are still offered, including through dreaming, a special condition by which to reestablish emotional contact with their most intimate selves and their significant others, with the most privileged Other being the therapist as an active listener and humane companion throughout the analytic journey.

In this way, the psychotic patient, as an occasional dreamer, is recognized as having a most fundamental yet idiosyncratic embodied mind. He or she is progressively given, by means of the analytic process itself, both the protected time and the protective space to simply be, to come to exist as a living human being with regard to the mentality and physicality of his or her self. In other words, psychotic individuals will ultimately come to sense their own body not simply as a disorganized, corrupted, broken, or even dead thing but as a dreaming body, that is, a living container for the internal unconscious processing of crude chunks of self-experience and wordless relatedness to reference others.

This leads to the third role of dreaming, as interestingly envisaged by Berne (1969 [1957]), one that is particularly important in "digesting" emotions and therefore protecting individuals from psychotic breakdowns: "Many psychoses are preceded by a period of prolonged lack of sleep, and hence lack of opportunity to dream. It may be that the mass of 'undigested' emotions which results has some effect in bringing on the psychosis" (p. 136).

Berne did not, however, highlight a clear methodology for facilitating this digestive processing of emotions through dreaming, especially in relation to clinical work with psychotic patients. His view on the digestive function of dreams was, instead, further expanded in Bion's (1977 [1962]) *Learning from experience* and originally extended by Bion, through the concept of *reverie*, to include the individual's waking life:

> An emotional experience occurring in sleep ... does not differ from the emotional experience occurring during waking life in that the perceptions of the emotional experience have in both instances to be worked upon by alpha function before they can be used for dream thoughts. ... If the patient cannot transform his [raw sensory] emotional experiences into alpha-elements, he cannot dream. Alpha-function transforms sense impressions into alpha-elements which resemble, and may in fact be identical to, the visual images with which we are familiar in dreams, namely, the elements that Freud

198

regards as yielding their latent content [when interpreted in analysis or self-analysis]. ... Failure of alpha-function means that the patient cannot dream and therefore cannot sleep. [In as much as] alpha-function makes the [raw] sense impression ... available for conscious [thought] and dream-thought, the patient who cannot dream cannot go to sleep and cannot wake up. Hence the peculiar condition seen clinically when a psychotic patient behaves as if he were in precisely this state.

(pp. 6–7)

Therefore, if we take a more general Bionian perspective on structural pathology within a transactional analysis model of psychopathology, the excluding Child in active schizophrenia can be seen as responsible, on the one hand, for the evacuation through dreaming of beta-elements (C_1) in the presence of a primarily precarious alpha-function (i.e., P_1 exclusion). On the other hand, the Child of the schizophrenic patient happens to be an insufficient container for beta-elements coming from external reality and actual object relations, which cannot be properly digested as a result of the underdeveloped ability of A_1 to provide adequate alpha-function itself (i.e., a not-yet-integrated and traumatized A_1). Taking both of these aspects together, this leads to the patient's hallucinatory experiences and aberrant thoughts (delusions) in waking life as well as during sleep.

The therapy with Nathan (see section "Listening" in Chapter 6), the young fine arts student who presented with the onset of schizophrenia, provides a further clinical example that opens the way for a new perspective on the transactional analysis of dreams with psychotic patients.

Nathan began one of his sessions by saying,

(P = Patient, T = Therapist)

P: "I saw you in Leicester Square last night."
T: "Was I in Leicester Square last night?" I thought.

I was so dumbfounded by the patient's remark, really a question, that I needed a few minutes before I could be sure that I had not been in the city center the night before our session. In the meantime, however, I tried to take a bit of time to think over what I had actually done the previous day. I therefore asked why he had gone out the night before, and he replied simply, "I don't know." Finally, he added that he had spent the whole day at home playing on his PlayStation. I hypothesized that the patient had probably dreamed our meeting. Nevertheless, he continued to insist he had seen me in Leicester Square near the Tube station. He finally added that it had seemed really odd to him that I was still out and about at one in the morning. "Wow, that is downright impossible," I thought to myself. On an emotional level, however, I felt myself to be in some way inside the scene to which Nathan was inviting me: he and I meeting by chance in Leicester Square.

At that point in the session, I realized that Nathan was recounting a dream without being completely aware that it was a dream rather than an experience that had been "actually" lived. As a result, rather than confront him with reality in an attempt to show him that he was probably wrong, I chose instead to say something like, "Um, it's possible. Yes, it's possible that you saw me. In fact, Leicester Square is one of my favorite Tube stops." He answered me, immediately curious, "Really?" Yes, I told him honestly, it was true, that it was a Tube station I went to regularly either to get to Soho or to wander the narrow streets of Covent Garden or else to get off for the National Gallery, not to mention that Leicester Square itself was one of the regular rendezvous points for meeting friends and colleagues over the weekend. Nathan stayed silent, watching me with an expression that had become more melancholy. At that point, I involved him in something else that had actually happened to me and that had something to do with him and that place: "Do you know, when I left the Tube station, I came across a Cass Art shop that was right next to it." "Yes, I know it, it's a very good shop," he said to me with interest. I continued, "I often think about you, about your passion for drawing, whenever I see or go into a shop that sells art and design supplies." "Really?" he asked me in amazement. I told him emphatically yes, it was so, and I said that it had been a shame that we had not met the previous day.

The session ended by discussing his experiences of solitude, how his thoughts of being "constantly monitored" somehow by third parties, including me, were less disturbing in the evening and how he preferred to leave the house at night to go to places that are particularly crowded during the day so as to feel himself to still be part of the world.

At the next session, he brought me a pencil drawing he had done that depicted a glimpse of Leicester Square. He told me that the drawing was for me. And it is a little gift I cherish. For him it was important to know that I thought about him from one session to the next; for me, it was a reminder of him as a person, of his interests, hobbies, and artistic aspirations.

In Nathan's case, his dream seemed to unfold within the space created by the analytic dyad and, in particular, by the pre-egoic states deriving from his C_1. As such, his dream took the form of a fresh, unprocessed product requiring active digestion rather than intellectual interpretation. In such scenarios, the analyst is not only a witness (as in Chris's dream) and/or a participant (as in Alice's case) but is acting on the dream with his own reverie, as if he were in coauthorship with the patient. In other words, the analyst becomes an influencing presence by entering together with the patient into an oneiric dimension of reality: "The analyst participates in dreaming the dreams that the patient is unable to dream on his own" (Ogden, 2005, p. 5). What remains with the analyst is, however, in Berne's (1969 [1957]) view, the ultimate responsibility for guiding the patient through the understanding of reality:

One of the most important things in life is to understand reality and to keep changing our images to correspond to it, for it is our images which determine our actions and feelings, and the more accurate they are the easier it will be for us to attain happiness and stay happy in an ever-changing world where happiness depends in large part on other people.

(p. 46)

Nathan's account of his "dreamy world" further corroborates the view that the psychotic atmosphere—which is normally found in active schizophrenia—originates in the person's emotionally charged sensate perceptions, almost invariably coupled with more or less unconscious unilateral interpretations of potentially any object of experience. This includes one's own body and bodily functions, other people's words and observable behaviors, things, animals, physical (also natural) as well as social events, and dreams themselves, regardless of the more conventional categories of time and space.

Conversely, and still from the patient's perspective, overcoming a psychotic crisis—including through the multiple meanings unfolding from dream analysis—is less about coming to understand what "reality" in general truly is or means. Instead, breaking through psychosis is about becoming a real person, which ultimately leads the individual to discover (or rediscover) and responsibly deal with the persistence in life of two main dimensions of experience: the inner world and the outside world and their respective complexities and nonconscious interrelations. This discovery usually comes with the later acknowledgment, by the patient experiencing psychosis, that both of these worlds are populated by many Other(s), that is, by whomever is able to leave historical traces (even scars) of their passage in his or her life, psyche, and body in the culture and communities to which the person belongs and in which he or she lives.

In other words, because the world of psychosis is one in which any forms of true alterity can barely survive, becoming a real person means welcoming the Other(s) and otherness both within and without ourselves. Thus even "dreaming together," by both the patient and the analyst, clearly leads to forming an "I and You" and a "We" relatedness. It means that something is unequivocally happening—bodily, psychologically, relationally, socially—between two or more real persons coming together in the here and now of the therapeutic encounter. However, in my view, dreaming together requires much effort from the analyst in trusting both his or her own and the patient's unconscious in order for old tensions to be released, previous fractures to pave the way for more constructive future directions, new emotions to be exchanged, new meanings to be cocreated, and ultimately more humanity to be shared and comprehended within the space and time offered by the analytic setting.

In summary, in more general terms, the art of interpreting dreams in psychotic processes moves on from the fundamental consideration that the manifest dream is the "real" dream for the patient. The second methodological step is to engage emotionally, through countertransference, with the role (i.e., part, object) unconsciously assigned to the analyst within the transference relationship as it is (re)dramatized in the patient's dream. A third methodological step in dreamwork with schizophrenic patients ultimately requires the analyst to "dream together with the patient" (Ehebald, 1981). This involves entering a somewhat oneiric bipersonal (or even multipersonal) arena (Ferro, 1999) or contacting an unconscious intersubjective "analytic third" (Ogden, 1994) in which very early non(yet)conscious and unconscious (through contamination and exclusion) memories become integrated into new meanings according to the patient's emotional history, the history of the therapeutic process, and the here and now of the analytic session.

Dreaming the analysis

By "dreaming the analysis," I am referring to welcoming actual dreams as they emerge during analytic therapy, dreams in which either the psychotic patient or the analyst has dreamed about the other and/or about the analytic session(s).

When a psychotic patient dreams about his or her analyst and is able to communicate this in the therapy room, I consider it a turning point in the analytic process: a new psychological space between reality and fantasy has been created. I think of this as a transitional space in which the dreamer's (patient, analyst, or both) imagination takes over autistic phantasy, allowing the self to come imaginatively to life and then to speak his or her own voice in the presence of a new significant other. It is the analyst's responsibility to then assist the patient in further developing this capacity for dreaming reality— including the reality of one's self and the other during the therapeutic encounter—and therefore for starting (or continuing) to think symbolically through visual imagery.

For example, during one of my visits to her house, Anisha—the patient I previously described who was the daughter of the Indian diplomat with a degree from Princeton in Indian literature—unexpectedly recounted a dream that heralded a new phase in our work together.

(P = Patient, T = Therapist)

P: "Last night I had a dream ... about the two of us and a fox."

T: "A fox?"

P: "Yes."

T: "I sense that you're worried, is that right?"

P: "In Indian culture, dreams represent a time of being in between, a bridge linking the past, the present, and the future."

202

T: "Wow, what a fascinating idea, it seems to contain the wisdom of centuries."[Long silence].

T: "But what was your dream, Anisha?"

P: "You and I are here, at my house. This room is completely empty and everything around me seems utterly surreal. You sit, as you usually do, opposite me, on that armchair, exactly where you are sitting now. But we aren't alone. A fox is walking round the room, and at a certain point it comes toward my armchair. I am petrified with fear. With a silent leap, it jumps on me, and I find it on my lap, as quiet as a tame wolf. I close my eyes. I feel it climbing up the back of the chair to settle like a living fur collar around my neck. I am stunned and curious about its presence. I feel its warmth around my face. When I open my eyes, you're no longer there, you've left."

Both Anisha and I immediately fell prey to a plethora of interpretative suggestions about the dream. The first association—also one of the fairly obvious ones—that immediately came to my mind, and which I shared with the her, had to do with the fact that the fox, and the wolf, somehow reminded one of the night, and, therefore, of the same unconscious, dreamy nocturnal dimension of existence. For Anisha, the fox was, instead, an embodiment of intuition, shrewdness, and cunning. We both concluded that it (the fox) in other respects represented the essence of our therapy, which was made up of impressions and led by sensations, poetic evocations, twilight photos and images, in an atmosphere of intimacy and semidarkness, even in broad daylight. We were both then struck by the element of surprise evoked by the, so to speak, "tame" attitude of the fox to the point where Anisha asked, rhetorically, the question that the little prince of Antoine de Saint Exupéry (1995 [1943], p. 76) asks his fox: "What does it mean—tame?" And when all was said and done, our analysis up to that moment had been a kind of reciprocal taming that resulted in the creation of a connection.

However, there was something that this analysis of Anisha's dream had not touched on, and that was the element of the temporal bridge with the future to which she herself had referred in her story. It was something I had not considered up to that point apart from on a merely cultural level primarily associated with the view of dreams in Indian culture. That dream was, in reality, the beginning of a goodbye that happened about six months later when I was given the opportunity of furthering my professional career in Switzerland. The dream concluded with my disappearance from the scene but also with the comfort of a new presence, the fox, now a living part of Anisha's clothing and, therefore, also of her ego. It was a bridge between the internal world and the external world, between darkness and light, between dreams and reality, between what had been and what was not yet. We returned a number of times to this dream, which accompanied and kept watch over our analysis up until the final session.

Whenever I return to London and I encounter one of the foxes that prowl at night around certain city boroughs, I cannot help thinking again of Anisha's dream and her troubled history. And in these situations I also like to imagine that Anisha herself has become a fox and that she is seeking someone else to tame.

On the other hand, as a transactional analyst, whenever I dream about one of my psychotic patients, before communicating the experience directly to him or her in the analytic setting, I request supervision. I do this for two reasons. First, I often daydream about my patients, their lives, their relationships, and their futures, sometimes in the middle of a session with the patient. Second, and closely linked to the first, is that any confession of a daydream about a psychotic patient, especially if that dream has not been properly digested, may have a traumatic effect on the already fragile ego of that patient and compromise, among other things, the therapeutic alliance.

The case of Mr Blake, as the reader can probably imagine, required a fair amount of self-analysis and supervision on my part because of the powerful projective inductions he was able to generate and that put a strain on my countertransference at a bodily-emotional level. The following is an excerpt of a dream I had about him that I think explains, not only in that specific case, the informative power of dream processes regarding both the pathology of these patients and the cotransferential processes in the analytic relationship. The resulting therapeutic effects often, in order to be useful, require a second digestion through supervision. The dream I describe here disturbed me greatly on an emotional level.

> I am in my flat in Herne Hill on a rare sunny day, and I am going out to take a walk in the park. The doorbell rings, and when I open the front door, I find five uniformed police officers before me. They ask me to say who I am and tell me that they have orders to carry out a "persecuzione" (persecution) (wow, what a slip of the tongue, I meant a "p-e-r-q-u-i-s-i-z-i-o-n-e" or search) in my back garden behind the house. I am completely speechless, as if paralyzed by the request, which is, in fact, an order. At that point, four of them storm into the flat while one of the police officers, the only one wearing a pair of dark glasses, remains outside the house to guard the entrance. His figure worries me, but I don't know why at that point. They order me to open the back door and to wait behind them. Two of them go toward the bottom of the lawn where there is a little gazebo where I usually pile up my gardening tools. I try to ask them what is going on, but they order me to be quiet. I ask who sent them and they tell me again to be silent. Two female police officers stand near me, and I see them start talking to one another in low voices. I hear them laugh softly and make derogatory comments about me. I think it is some-thing like, "He's so stupid," "But how could he? What an idiot!"

"Who knows what the neighbors will say about it." I feel deep irritation watching those two women talking to each other, more like a
couple of old gossips than police officers. I ask them what they are
talking about. They answer sarcastically that they are not obliged to
tell me anything. I feel increasingly distressed, and I move toward the
other two police officers near the gazebo. The scene I come upon is
disturbing: from a black bag buried in the dust, I see the two officers
take out the remains of a body, perhaps more than one. A police
officer looks at me and tells me that the corpses are all the headless
bodies of little children. In the garden there is no sign of the heads
that belong to these bodies. I am overcome with anguish. I begin to
shout at the top of my voice that I don't know anything about it, that
I have nothing to do with it, and I run away. No one stops me. As I
leave through the front door, I encounter the police officer in the
sunglasses. I throw myself astonished into his arms, almost as if I'm
seeking protection. He receives me warmly, and then in a gentle voice
tells me to calm down, not to think about it. "How can I not think
about it?" I cry. When I burst into tears, he grabs my face violently
and kisses me firmly on the mouth. At that point, I wake up with my
heart in my mouth. I am covered in sweat. As I cannot get back to
sleep, while I am still upset and disoriented, as if I have really lived
the whole event, my first thought goes to that last scene, to the
Caucasian police officer with the sunglasses who, however, I immediately associate with my dark-skinned patient, Mr Blake. At that
point, I write down on a piece of paper everything I have attempted
to recount here.

I set up a supervision session almost two weeks after this dream. I remember reporting fairly decisively to my supervisor a series of reflections made
retrospectively in expectation of our supervision, including the following: (1)
it was a countertransference dream; (2) I assumed this because of the unconscious association between the police officer's sunglasses and those of Mr
Blake, known to attend his analytic sessions wearing a pair of black Ray
Bans; (3) I had noticed a reversal of roles, in the sense that the one who was
"persecuted" in the dream was me and not the patient because it happened in
my own home, and it was me who was forced to scour the back of my garden
(figuratively speaking, the "past" and the "unconscious"); (4) the dismembered bodies of the children, of whose murder I felt implicitly accused in
the dream, represented parts of an "infantile" alter ego of the patient's
mother. Indeed, in the past the patient had often showed particularly violent
thoughts, impulses, and on two occasions, even actual violence toward his
mother and, later on, toward one of his female teachers. As evidence for these
reflections, I continued to provide anamnestic facts about my patient. I concluded in the presence of my supervisor that this was a dream in which I had

been able to feel exactly what Mr Blake had probably experienced in the analytic relationship: (1) feeling persecuted, even by me; (2) having to submit to me dragging out (figuratively into the "sunlight") what lay "at the back" of his mind, including derogatory voices and paranoia about his neighbors; and (3) having presumed homosexual tendencies of which he probably was not aware and that led to feeling a certain attraction toward me.

However, my self-analysis left out at least two aspects that I had somehow omitted from my reflections and that, in fact, became an unexpected focus for the supervision: (1) my total passivity in relation to the presumed homosexual attraction of the police officer with the glasses, whom I had identified in my semiawake state as Mr Blake; and (2) the fact that the police officer with the glasses had white skin and was not dark like my patient. To these thoughts, my supervisor provocatively added the whispered gossip of the "two female police officers very close to me." In an attempt to find other possible meanings for these new elements, my supervisor suggested that we linger a little longer on my emotional and bodily experiences in those precise moments in the dream, despite the fact that I deemed myself to be merely the mirror to Mr Blake's drama. "Where is your part, or your parts, in all of this, in this dream?" my supervisor asked, leaving me in more doubt than ever. In a subsequent supervision session several days after the first one, we returned to the final unexpressed aspects of the dream. After an initial sense of bewilderment, while I was still trying to piece together the previous session, my supervisor asked me gently whether this dream was a way of "convincing him" of the fact that he (i.e., the supervisor), too, had an erotic attraction to me and I to him. I remember having received his comment with a dense silence, but something of my transference, which had not emerged from the dream, somehow imposed itself onto the supervision session.

Therefore, during the supervision session, I made an embarrassing confession:

> When I was 7 years old, I was hit by a car in the main square of my village. It was 25 April 1987, the day when Italy marks the anniversary of its liberation from Fascism and Nazi occupation. I had gone to buy the newspaper for my father, who was ill in bed that day. I was feeling proud of myself for doing this, both important and energized. Unfortunately, on my way back, I crossed the road carelessly, without looking to my left. When I saw the car coming, it was already too late, and I ended up with my left leg halfway under the front wheel. The driver put the brakes on with such a loud screech that my mother looked out of the window of the house and was left shocked and literally paralyzed by the accident. I was quickly taken to hospital and underwent an emergency operation for a fracture of my tibia that had partly damaged a tendon, thus threatening to leave me crippled for life. I remember that while I was in hospital, the only

person I wanted with me every day was my father. I stubbornly refused to be visited by my mother, who was upset at my reaction, and I didn't ask to see my beloved little sister for several weeks. When I returned home, I felt as if I were starting a new life, as if it was not my real house, and my parents and my sister were not my real family. Fortunately, this distressing situation resolved itself over time with a lot of effort and love shown every day by my family. Nevertheless, I remember that during the worst of this both physical and mental distress, every night, when the lights were turned out, I went silently to the bed where my parents slept and secretly kissed my father on the mouth. I think I did this for several months almost every evening, and then more rarely for a few years, without ever finding up to now a "true" explanation for why I did it.

It was only at this point in the supervision, after having shared a very traumatic experience from my past, that the dream about Mr Blake acquired a new and totally unexpected perspective: (1) the Caucasian police officer with the sunglasses, who had remained outside the scene of the search, reminded me of my father, who for some reason (probably only his illness?) had not come to the place of the "accident"; (2) something about my infant relationships with female significant others, especially my mother, appeared as if dismembered, dead, hidden somewhere and for a long time; and (3) the two female police officers who were chatting to each other instead of listening to me (or even helping me) reminded me of two of my female neighbors, who also came the day of my accident in place of my mother, but who were generally more interested in disapproving of everything and gossiping than maintaining cordial and supportive relationships.

As for being a countertransference dream about Mr Blake, it actually contained elements of my own personal history that were not relevant to or were frankly misleading about what the patient was experiencing in the analytic present (transference from the analyst onto the patient). But that is just what the supervision gradually sought to unravel, in the process revealing my unconscious defenses as an analyst, defenses that threatened to tarnish a shared and shareable reading of the patient's experiences as they had been dramatized in the dream.

In light of these final considerations, what remained of the dream—without the unconscious contribution of my transference—seemed to take on a new form, which I expressed to my supervisor in pretty much these words: "What would have happened to the interpretation of this dream if the perspective of I-dreamer had been not that of I-narrator but rather that of the Caucasian police officer with the dark sunglasses?" Basically, I thought, could there be another plausible and perhaps less Machiavellian hypothesis than the first one? I am the white-skinned police officer-analyst, wearing the dark lenses of my patient, dissociating myself, rather like he does, from traumatic experiences that belong not only to his personal history but also to mine.

Following this alternative hypothesis, the "I-police officer with the sunglasses" would therefore have been complicit both in the "perquisizione-persecuzione" (search-persecution) of the patient but also responsible for a homoerotic seduction of the patient himself in an attempt to stop the madness. *Mutatis mutandis* this was beginning to echo what I was experiencing in the analytic relationship with Mr Blake. My interventions aimed at retracing the mostly painful chapters of his past had been experienced by the patient as inquisitorial. My unnatural calm in the relationship concealed an unexpressed fear of being attacked, at times physically, by the patient. In some situations, this fear had been, by means of a projective identification by me, perceived as an eroticization of certain behaviors by the patient during the sessions. The initial hypothesis, in which I had analyzed him as having latent homosexual tendencies toward me, was revealed—in light of what emerged from the supervision and with the progression of the analysis itself—to be without foundation and not in line with the patient's psychobiographical experiences. The patient's psychodevelopmental history showed, in fact, how he had seen every expectation of love and protection by his paternal Parent powerfully and repeatedly betrayed. This prevented Mr Blake from accepting, particularly at the start of the analysis, even the most minimal demonstration of "masculine" love and protection by me in the analytic relationship. In actual fact, the patient acknowledged nourishing profoundly homophobic feelings, even toward me, and, at the same time, while he was able to establish relationships with people of the opposite sex, these relationships ended up becoming highly disturbing because the women he was with were unconsciously superimposed onto the mad, ineffectual, emotionally toxic maternal alter ego.

As the aforementioned examples show, supervision about dreams is particularly beneficial in every situation in which the analyst experiences his or her own particularly powerful bodily-emotional transference. Such transference, among other things, is an indicator of a high permeability and precariousness of the (inter)egoic boundaries between the analyst and the schizophrenic patient.

References

Abraham, K. (1955). Dreams and myths: A study in folk-psychology. In K. Abraham, H. & M. D. Abraham (Eds.) *Clinical papers and essays on psycho-analysis* (pp. 153–209). London: The Hogarth Press and the Institute of Psychoanalysis. (Original work published 1909)

Berne, E. (1969). *A layman's guide to psychiatry and psychoanalysis.* London: Andre Deutsch. (Original work published 1957)

Berne, E. (1975). *What do you say after you say hello? The psychology of human destiny.* London: Corgi. (Original work published 1972)

Bion, W. R. (1977). *Learning from experience.* London: William Heinemar. (Original work published 1962) de Saint Exupéry, A. (1995). *The little prince.* Ware: Wordsworth Editions. (Original work published 1943)

Ehebald, U. (1981). Überlegungen zur Einschätzung des manifesten Traumes [Considerations for the assessment of the manifest dream]. In U. Ehebald & F. W. Eikhoff, (Eds.), *Humanität und Technik in der Psychoanalyse: Jahrbuch der Psychoanalyse* (Booklet 6, pp. 81–100). Bern: Hans Huber.

Fairbairn, W. R. D. (1952). *An object-relations theory of the personality.* New York, NY: Basic Books.

Ferro, A. (1999). *The bi-personal field: Experiences in child analysis.* London: Routledge.

Freud, S. (1953). The interpretation of dreams. In J. Strachey (Ed. & Trans.), *The standard edition of the complete psychological works of Sigmund Freud* (Vol. 4, pp. 1–338; Vol. 5, pp. 339–630). London: Hogarth Press. (Original work published 1900)

Klein, M. (1975). *Narrative of a Child Analysis.* New York, NY: Delacorte. (Original work published in 1961).

Klein, M. (1997). *The psycho-analysis of children.* London: Vintage. (Original work published 1932).

Ogden, T. H. (1994). The analytic third: Working with intersubjective clinical facts. *International Journal of Psychoanalysis*, 75, 3–20.

Ogden, T. H. (2005). *This art of psychoanalysis: Dreaming undreamt dreams and interrupted cries.* London: Routledge.

Tangolo, A. E. (2015). Group imago and dreamwork in group therapy. *Transactional Analysis Journal*, 45, 179–190.

10

DON'T HIDE THE MADNESS

Undoubtedly, schizophrenia both distorts and fragments the usual experience of one's self as well as the perception one unceasingly creates of other people, the world, and life in general. It dramatically disrupts the feeling one has of the ordinary. However, when someone asks me directly what schizophrenia actually is or means, I tend to answer that it is essentially a relational fact. It is relational because it does not belong to the single individual but to one's subjective experience of feeling strange, estranged, and even alienated. Invariably, this is in relation to someone else and/or physical objects, places, animals, and nature, all of which become infused by the self with special, in some cases rather worrying, significance or connectedness. It is also a "fact" because it starts off, and then tends to persist, as a relational experience, that is, an experience that originates in the individual's most troubled relationships with real significant others. This more existential perspective on psychosis clearly echoes the ideas proposed by Berne (1975 [1961]) and other original thinkers and clinicians such as Laing (1959) and, more recently, Bollas (2015). Their works stem from the more general view that a psychotic breakdown could be a potentially creative and transformative response to real relational struggles that the psychotic person faced—and usually continues to face—in the family and microsocial milieu and in the absence of corrective relationships (and identifications) outside the family. Thus, psychosis is understandable and meaningful from within patients' relational and social (including familial) vicissitudes.

For these reasons, there is no such thing as a "schizophrenic ego" in the same way that there is no "diabetic ego" or "arthritic ego" and so on. Instead, there is an individual with schizophrenia or diabetes or arthritis—the person, therefore, as subject before any other reduction, definition, or diagnostic category. And this must be our fundamental priority: preserving the real self, that most vital and irreducible part of our being-in-relation-to-the-Other and Otherness, which survives even the most severe mental and physical suffering and which I have called here the "naked self."

But let us return to schizophrenia and its etymology, deriving as it does from the apposition of two words from Greek: the verb σκίζειν, meaning "to split, divide," and -φρενία, which is related to φρήν φρενός, meaning "mind." Therefore, "schizophrenia" is a way of saying, incorrectly, "divided mind." And it is a way of not saying many other things, such as what schizophrenia ultimately brings to the person who suffers from it, including the ability to feel, imagine, think, act, and relate to others and the surrounding world.

In essence, schizophrenia makes us return to being, or perhaps makes us more than usually unprepared for life, for everyday life, especially for living among other people. A patient of nearly 50 with schizophrenia, whom I met several years ago during my first years of specialist training, described in a few poignant words what suffering from schizophrenia meant for him: "I feel like a grown-up child, grown-up certainly, but still a child." I think his words sum up the essence of the schizophrenic experience, one that we may all face on our journey of life in an equally sensitive epoch of our development as human beings: the transition from adolescence to adulthood. This phase of our life story harkens back to another transition in the life of every individual: from childhood to early adolescence. It is no coincidence that schizophrenia mainly affects those periods in our life in which we have the chance to demonstrate to ourselves, and those around us, whether we are ready for the present and the future, for what we do not yet know, for the unknown, for encountering the new others who await us just beyond our family group, for what life in general can bring us in terms of suffering but also joy.

Schizophrenia is, in other words, an attempt to move forward in life, trying to respond to personal, family, and social urges in the present moment and doing so despite the unshakable fear of relationships with others, despite the fear of the future, the fear of suffering, and, paradoxically, the fear of joy.

Thoughts not shared with others become thoughts that others do not share, that is, thoughts that others do not understand and ultimately do not accept. Thoughts like these are given the name "delusions," that is, ideas that deviate from others' thoughts and move away from other persons. Feelings not shared with others become "hallucinations," that is, feelings that others do not perceive. Little by little, we stop having healthy illusions about reality and also stop imagining and even really hoping—which is more terrible still—that someone is knocking on our door, is coming to seek us out, is there for us.

The body can also send signals that the person does not understand, thereby adding anguish about his or her physical as well as mental integrity. People sometimes become frozen in their own movements, often silent and even mute, almost paralyzed by the fear of being in the world; or, conversely, they feel lost, in constant motion, although they do not have an actual goal or destination to reach.

In either case, the final outcome is alienation: the desperate renunciation of relating to others and therefore of the reality—which is, above all,

211

psychological—that others represent. This produces a deep pain that comes from the feeling of the lack of Others, a relational—and thus also intrapsychic—void that the person sometimes tries to fill with alcohol and drugs or behavior that endangers both themselves and other people.

But there is some good news. Schizophrenia, precisely because of the suffering it brings, paradoxically teaches us all at least two life lessons: first, that human beings' fundamental condition is that of depending on other human beings for their mental and physical health, and, therefore, for their own happiness; and second, we are not children for just a part of our lives, but a child part of us, our inner Child, hides behind this suffering and endlessly hopes to be sought, wanted, and ultimately found by others.

Consequently, when encountering a so-called "schizophrenic"—particularly in clinical and analytic settings—the true challenge is to find out where his or her "real" self or inner Child lives or hides, despite the psychosis. And most importantly, the challenge is to discover which parts, extensions, or fragments of the patient's actual self come to stay and even reside within ourselves. But that is the rub: to find the patient's real self, we need first to acknowledge that we ourselves live, from time to time, our own schizophrenic moments. We, too, generate, as our patients do, schizophrenic worries about other people, including families, friends, and work colleagues as well as, on a larger scale, other members of the society we live in and/or people belonging to other communities, such as foreigners or, even more simply, strangers.

In this way, every time we impose our ideas on others, every time we anticipate their thoughts, every time we claim to feel emotions in their place or force them to swallow an emotion that we ourselves do not know how to digest, we are colonizing other people's minds. Every time we stop being open-hearted with that person by shutting ourselves away in stubborn silence when we could, instead, talk, those times that we could admit to being weak and yet insist, at all costs, that we are strong out of pride, shame, fear, hate, or suffocating grudges that we hold within us, we are preventing both ourselves and others from being truly intimate with one another. All the times we make others wait an absurdly long time through our repeated absences, every time we lie or we attribute liability to third parties, saying they are at fault when we, ourselves, could shoulder the responsibility with just a modicum of courage and humility, those are times we are raising high walls between us and others. Every time we cast aspersions on others' behavior and their intentions because we would like them to be as we wish them to be, every time that we presume we can act on behalf of someone else when formulating a belief, a doubt, or, more to the point, when making a decision that does not primarily concern us, we are abusively intruding into someone's inner and relational world. Every time we use words as swords and call it "love," every time we caress someone when, in reality, we would like to hit them, especially when that person also depends on us for personal growth and differentiation and individuation as other-than-us, and particularly if this occurs in sensitive

212

phases of life such as the end of infancy and early adulthood—these are all the times when we are psychoticizing that person's experience of life. These are all the times when we are making other people live a terrible, schizophrenic moment, when we are fragmenting the continuity of their being and therefore their being, or becoming, a unique and inimitable individual.

If we really think about it, we all do these things every day, in a discontinuous, distracted, more or less surreptitious way. There are endless reasons we give ourselves or others, including our victims, for why we are behaving in such ways. Meanwhile, we are sowing seeds of madness capable of savagely occupying the mental and relational life of those who are at our side, in front of us, or under or even above us in age, role, authority, and power.

And, on the other hand, when we live our schizophrenic moments, we often discover with great terror how there are two main ways of escaping from reality—*in primis*, from the reality of the Other—that psychosis offers us: paranoia and body-mind dissociation. Paranoia allows us to pull off the miracle of transferring omnipotently the beam that has ended up in our own eye to the Other's eye, thereby transforming it into a bad eye, an "evil eye" against which we must guard ourselves with ceaseless suspicion and scorn. And dissociation is a kind of reduction into fragments and evacuation from the mind to elsewhere, outside one's own body, toward the body of the Other or toward other bodies, even those that are a long way away (such as the celestial bodies of Mr Blake) or an eclipse of the mind within one's own body (such as what happened to Abena), a hiding place for one's own self out in the open and in the presence of the Other.

To my patients—and others facing schizophrenia

The final words of this book are directed at you, my dear patient with schizophrenia, and at those who are by your side, with responsibility, at times with difficulty, and, at least I hope, with unconditional love. I want to end by opening my heart to you, never really knowing how to remain silent about the hopes for your welfare and mental and physical—and also spiritual—health, which I wish to nourish for you and your life today and tomorrow.

Avoid those who want to refute or ignore your delusional thoughts. Instead, find in those thoughts the multiple meanings they conceal. Talk out loud with a dear friend or confidant, a family member, better if also with a psychotherapist, about what at first sight seems bizarre to you or concerns you in some way. Share the emotional impact of these ideas, especially if they become insistent and keep recurring savagely in your mind. Set these thoughts free. Make sure they don't carry on being repeated in the same way. At the end of the day, act in such a way that another engages with you in what you most fear, your madness, so that your ego can blossom from the most precious frailties of your being.

Likewise, make a treasure of your solitude, which is not isolation but preparation for intimacy, for new encounters with others, for new returns home, refinding from time to time the Others of the past who reside within and without us.

Do not fear medication as long as it is prescribed by someone who is caring for you as a person. Always give yourself a good dose of art and music. Walk in nature. Learn, if you don't already, to love animals.

Avoid those who think you are someone whose feet aren't firmly fixed to the ground, a dreamer. Humanity needs those who know how to see reality with the eyes of a child, who know how to immerse themselves with wonder in nature because we are part of it in the same way that part of it is our psyche. The psyche is like a house: it is made of rooms and places and memories and feelings. And it is in the places we visit and in the people we meet. The only place that is relevant to us is, time and again, a piece of the other and therefore a piece of ourselves.

There is no need for you, therefore, to hallucinate reality, but instead reinvent it with illusions. Like poets—that's right, like poets—reduce hallucinations to illusions, bring fantasy back to where it started and where it is destined: to reality, which is always multiple and inexhaustible, as are other human beings that we meet, infinite despite their own finitude, each of them frail or injured in their own way and with interesting and resilient lives.

Remember also—and this is no small thing—that your psyche is also made of flesh and blood, of skin and viscera, of breaths, of tears and tremors, of laughter and intentions, and it feeds on sights and sounds and smells and flavors and a handshake. So look after your body. It knows everything. It is the extension of your being and of your whole mind, conscious and nonconscious. It is the proof that we are also the legacy of someone else who has come before us. It is the proof that we are not enough by or for ourselves, that we have insurmountable limits. Not even extending our gaze helps us to see ourselves in our entirety, because entirety means multiplicity and therefore infinity. And thus it means allowing many others to view us from many angles and from many perspectives in order to capture the infinity that is in us and in others.

Having a body also means coming face to face with our imperfections and injuries on our skin. It means remembering. It means recognizing that we do not decide everything ourselves and that deciding something means bringing in discontinuities with the past. It means personally welcoming in new traumas and new crises with painful respect for the suffering they bring. Our body is also the substance of which our aspirations are made, that is, the acts of drawing to us, thus of aspiring and respiring what is around us. Our body reminds us that the greatest aspirations are others, nature, the cosmos, and that we can only take it in as well as release it a little at a time. In being a body, we are truly naked and innocent, like newborn babies and children who chew reality into small pieces and chunks, learning with effort to digest life a bit at a time, contributing to the continual discovery of themselves, joining in with the play—that's right, the play—in the wonder and the mystery of being and of being in relation to others.

So look after this "naked self" that is hidden within all of us and who always yearns for the Other. And remember that we all, from infancy, have an innate need to pretend reality, that is, create it and share it with others. Every one of us needs an "I" and a "you" and a "we"—a multiplicity of faces—in the same way that we need a multitude of seasons and colors and melodies and different places to give meaning to our everyday existence and to make us distinct from and therefore recognizable to each other.

Be wary of anyone who wants to view your schizophrenia as a mystical experience, an almost supernatural gift, and watch out too for anyone who wants to reduce it to a mythical experience, almost legendary and therefore false. Talk, instead, about your truth, albeit in the midst of suffering.

Finally, I want to tell you that, while I do not live it personally—although I do at times and in the occasional dream—I know that if you could lessen this suffering, or if you could at least alleviate it a little, you would do so because you are a human being just like me. As such you are called to life and death and, in the meantime, to live in this world with responsibility, hope, and joy. And, if you want, also with me by your side.

References

Berne, E. (1975). *Transactional analysis in psychotherapy: A systematic individual and social psychiatry.* London: Souvenir Press. (Original work published 1961)

Bollas, C. (2015). *When the sun bursts: The enigma of schizophrenia.* New Haven, CT: Yale University Press.

Laing, R. D. (1959). *The divided self: An existential study in sanity and madness.* London: Penguin Books.

INDEX

216

For Product Safety Concerns and Information please contact our EU
representative GPSR@taylorandfrancis.com
Taylor & Francis Verlag GmbH, Kaufingerstraße 24, 80331 München, Germany

www.ingramcontent.com/pod-product-compliance
Lightning Source LLC
Chambersburg PA
CBHW050422280326
41932CB00013BA/1956

9 780367 148423